PERSONAL CONSTRUCT THERAPY: A HANDBOOK

Developments in Clinical Psychology

Glenn R. Caddy, series editor
Nova University

MMPI-168 Codebook, by Ken R. Vincent, Iliana Castillo, Robert I. Hauser, H. James Stuart, Javier A. Zapata, Cal K. Cohn, and Gregory O'Shanick, 1984

Integrated Clinical and Fiscal Management in Mental Health: A Guidebook, by Fred Newman and James Sorensen, 1986

The Professional Practice of Psychology, edited by Georgiana Shick Tryon, 1986

Clinical Applications of Hypnosis, edited by Frank A. DePiano and Herman C. Salzberg, 1986

Full Battery Codebook, by Ken R. Vincent, 1987

Development in the Assessment and Treatment of Addictive Behaviors, edited by Ted D. Nirenberg, 1987

Feminist Psychotherapies, edited by Mary Ann Douglas and Lenore E. Walker, 1988

Child Multimodal Therapy, by Donald B. Keat II, 1990

Psychophysiology for Clinical Psychologists, by Walter W. Surwillo, 1990

Strategic Health Planning: Methods and Techniques Applied to Marketing and Management, by Allen D. Spiegel and Herbert H. Hyman, 1991

Behavioral Medicine: International Perspectives (Vol. 1–3), edited by D.G. Byrne and Glenn R. Caddy, 1992

The MMPI: A Contemporary Normative Study of Adolescents, edited by Robert C. Colligan and Kenneth P. Offord, 1992

Adult-Child Research and Experience, by Robert E. Haskell, 1993

Reprogramming Pain, by Barry Bittman, 1995

Personal Construct Therapy: A Handbook, by Linda L. Viney, 1996

PERSONAL CONSTRUCT THERAPY: A HANDBOOK

Linda L. Viney
University of Wollongong

Ablex Publishing Corporation
Norwood, New Jersey

Printed in the United States of America

Viney, Linda L.
Personal construct therapy : a handbook / Linda L. Viney.
p. cm. — (Developments in clinical psychology)
Includes bibliographical references and index.
ISBN 1-56750-229-6 (cloth)
1. Personal construct therapy. I. Title. II. Series.
[DNLM: 1. Psychotherapy. 2. Personal Construct Theory. WM 420 V738p 1996]
RC489.P46V563 1996
616.89'14—dc20
DNLM/DLC
for Library of Congress 96-19463
CIP

Ablex Publishing Corporation
355 Chestnut Street
Norwood, New Jersey 07648

This book is dedicated to my clients and to the students
of psychotherapy who have worked with me,
from both of whom I have learned so much.

Contents

I

LEARNING A NEW THERAPY

1

The Need for Personal Construct Therapy

I want to begin this book by telling the story of why I decided to write it. As a therapist and someone who trains other therapists, I am often asked: "But how do you do therapy?" It therefore seems appropriate to write a book that provides some of the answers. I have also found that I cannot merely describe the "doing" of therapy, but that I want to place it in a context that is both personal and conceptual. This book, then, is at least as much about me as it is about my clients, self-centered as that may sound. It is also about the ideas that I use to make sense of both my clients and myself. In it I present an approach, *personal construct therapy,* that works for me and my clients. It can work for you too. In this chapter, I introduce some personal construct therapy ideas and compare them with the ideas of other therapies. I also review the research that indicates the power of this therapy.

THE ROLE OF IDEAS IN PSYCHOTHERAPY

How can I as a therapist make sense of my clients without an integrated set of propositions to guide me in my thinking? I cannot. Neither can I assess and understand my clients without these ideas, nor set therapeutic goals with them without this assessment, nor monitor whether those goals are achieved. What about myself as a therapist? I cannot conceptualize, assess, set goals for, and monitor my own contributions to therapy without ideas. I introduce, too, the basic ideas of personal construct therapy and contrast them with those of the psychodynamic and cognitive-behavioral therapies. Some strategies of personal construct therapy are also contrasted here with those of other therapies.

SOME CONSTRUCTIVIST IDEAS

The constructivist assumptions underlying personal construct therapy are both complex and thought provoking and I attempt to do them justice in Chapters 2 and 3. Here I present a summary of seven of them:

1. People use constructs, or personal meanings, to make sense of what happens to them not only in the past and present, but also in the future. These constructs function together in a system of constructs.
2. The constructs, or interpretations and predictions, of any one individual are unique because they have been created from successive interpretations of the events experienced by that person.
3. Some constructs can be shared by groups of people.
4. Finding out about people's constructs enables understanding of their actions, both by themselves and by others in interaction.
5. The systems of constructs of psychologically healthy people are useful to them, if they provide the means to interpret and predict events, but not when they passively reflect those events.
6. When people's construct systems receive validation, or confirmation, indicating successful interpretation and prediction, it is positive emotion that is likely to result. However, when they are invalidated, or disconfirmed, indicating unsuccessful interpretation and prediction, it is negative emotion that they experience.
7. All constructs can be revised or replaced by other better interpretations or predictions.

If you find that some of these terms are unfamiliar, the glossary in which they are defined at the end of this book will help.

You should also find useful a diagramatic representation of how people's construct system function in the context of the world in which they live. Such a diagram can be found in Figure 1. This figure shows some of the processes by which the constructs or personal meanings of any one of us are tested and retested in our daily lives. Events that have been experienced by us, when we compare them, lead to personal constructs, which we then use to understand our own actions and those of other people. These constructs, then, come together in a construct system. This system has its own core and peripheral constructs but they are not considered here because I examine the structure of that system in a later chapter of this book. However, as Figure 1 shows, our construct systems are used to interpret and predict events. When our constructs are acted on, and validated or confirmed, they are retained

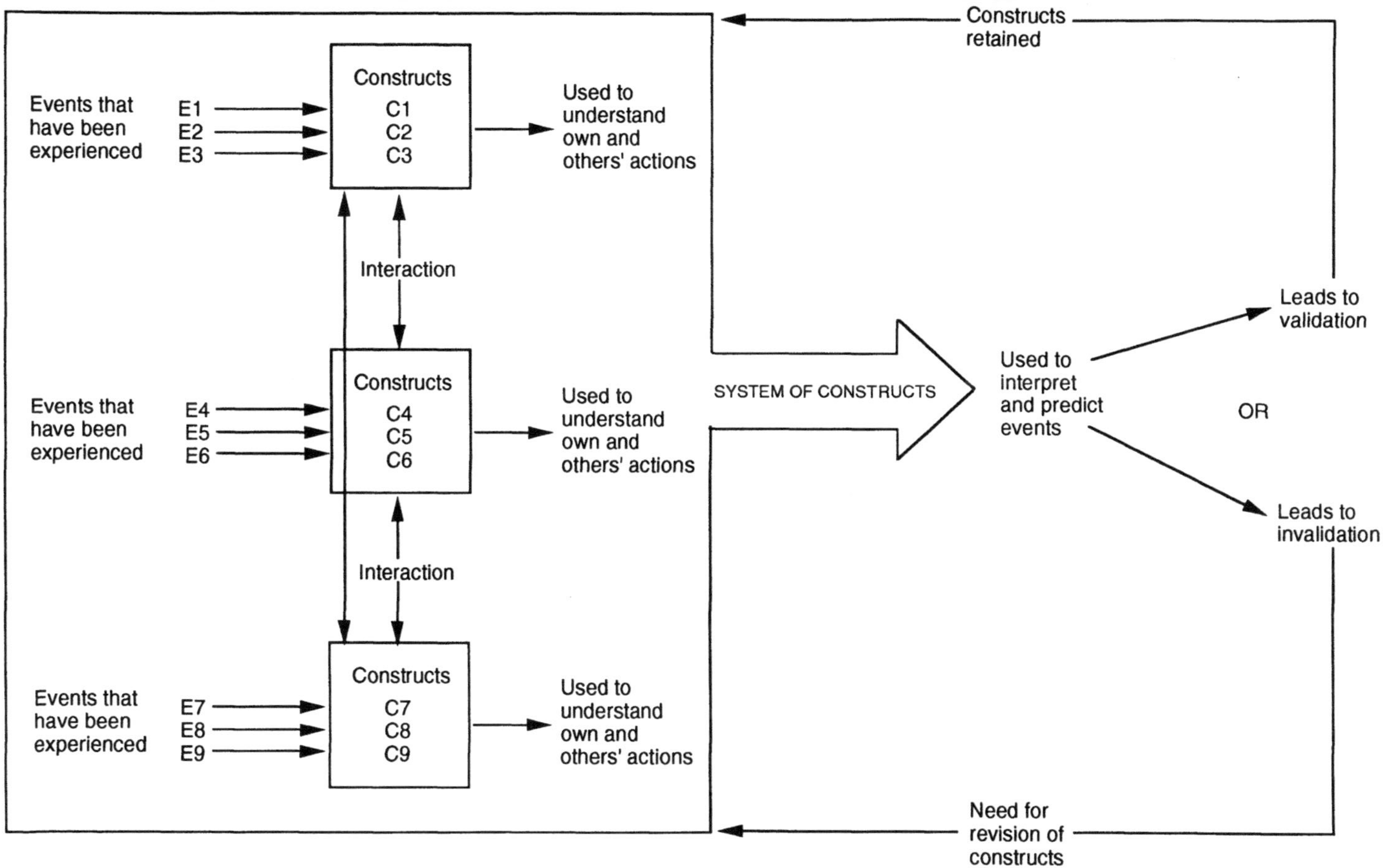

FIGURE 1. The Functioning of a System of Personal Constructs in its Context.

in our construct system. When they are acted on, and not validated or disconfirmed, we need to revise them. These processes occur for all psychologically healthy people. It is when some of these processes are blocked that clients find their way to us.

PERSONAL CONSTRUCT THERAPY

As a personal construct therapist, I see both my clients and myself as construers or makers of meaning (Kelly, 1955). Our constructs are built up, from a lifetime of experiences, into construct systems in which each construct has an impact, not just of itself but as it influences and is influenced by other constructs in the system (Bannister & Fransella, 1985). My clients, then, although they are usually not aware of this, come to therapy because their construct systems do not enable them to effectively interpret current events and predict future ones (Dalton & Dunnett, 1993). They will have indirect evidence of this through the negative emotions they experience. This lack of effectiveness could be because of the content of their constructs or because of the way they apply them. As a therapist, I bring my own construct system to therapy (Epting, 1984). I use that system to find ways to help clients test the problematic parts of their construct systems, as well as to monitor my own contribution to therapy. My goals, broadly, are to help my clients arrive at better interpretations and predictions of events and a wider range of choices in the future (Viney, 1994; Winter, 1990).

SOME RESEARCH EVALUATING PERSONAL CONSTRUCT THERAPY

The most recent review of this research in a prestigious international journal (Neimeyer, 1993) examined studies in which the outcomes of this therapy are contrasted with those of other therapies, as well as studies of client factors which can be linked with good therapeutic outcomes. The conclusion from this review was that there is good evidence for the effectiveness of this therapy but that more research in this area needs to be carried out. Another recent review (Winter, 1992), traced the 30-year history of this research, identifying among the many case studies of its effective application six independent groups of sample-based studies of outcome. This reviewer, too, noted the generally positive results of this research, whereas calling for more studies to be carried out, especially to show to which clients the different forms of this therapy are best suited. He also observed that there has been good research-based support for the applications of personal construct ideas in group therapy. This research is described in Chapter 11 of this book.

One of the earliest studies of the outcomes of individual personal construct therapy compared it with rational-emotive therapy for clients who experienced anxiety about public speaking (Karst & Trexler, 1974). Both therapies reduced this specific anxiety to some extent but the impact of personal construct therapy was significantly greater. Another early study dealing with stutterers showed that personal construct therapy, in comparison with a behavioral therapy, help those stutterers better to develop meanings for themselves as nonstutterers and so they less often relapse back to their previous frequency of stuttering (Fransella, 1972). This finding of less relapse to old levels of stuttering has also been demonstrated in a more recent study (Evesham & Fransella, 1985). Another early study of therapy outcome that must be considered is based on the idea that clients who seem thought disordered may do so because of what has been described as serial invalidation or continuous disconfirmation of their construing over long periods of time (Bannister, Adams-Webber, Penn, & Radley, 1975). The effects of personal construct therapy based on this idea were compared with the use of all available techniques in a special treatment of clients diagnosed as having thought disorders in a psychiatric hospital. Neither treatment proved more effective than the other. However, recent developments in using constructivist ideas with difficult clients like these make it worthwhile to reevaluate the use of this therapy with them.

The bulk of the rigorous research evaluating the outcomes of personal construct therapy has been with clients who may be described as neurotic, rather than psychotic, or those experiencing stressful life events. An evaluation of its outcome with depressed clients showed not only more construing of themselves as closer to their ideal person and as more like others after therapy, but also more tolerant of logical inconsistencies in construing (Sheehan, 1985). Although pharmacological therapy for depression also showed the earlier two findings, it did not show the last of greater tolerance of inconsistencies. Personal construct therapy has also been shown to be successful with shy clients (McKain, Glass, Arnkoff, Sydnor-Greenberg, & Shea, 1988), and those who have eating disorders (Button, 1994).

There has also been research carried out to evaluate the impact of personal construct therapy on clients who are dealing with the severe stress of illness. An overview of this research is available (Viney, 1990). This group of researchers has contrasted the effects of personal construct therapy with those of a no-therapy control condition. With acutely ill, hospitalized clients, greater decreases have been shown in their anxiety, indirectly expressed anger, and helplessness not only immediately after therapy, but also 1 year later when they were compared with those with no treatment (Viney, Clarke, Bunn, & Benjamin, 1985a). A quicker physical recovery was also shown in these clients in the form of faster return to normal blood pressure and pulse rate (Viney, Clarke, Bunn, & Benjamin, 1985b). With elderly clients dealing with chronic illness, a significant impact on their anxiety and depression immediately after therapy has been shown (Viney, Benjamin, & Preston, 1989). A member of this research team also examined some of the validation processes of personal construct therapists, first with a single client (Viney, 1993) and later comparing the content of therapy sessions of personal construct therapists with those of four therapists using other types of therapies (Viney, 1994). Personal construct therapists proved to use more validation or confirmation than rational-emotive therapists but not more than client-centred therapists.

TWO OTHER PSYCHOTHERAPIES

The first approach to psychotherapy that was developed in any complexity is the psychodynamic one. It has of course influenced those that have come later. The cognitive-behavioral approaches, for example, developed at least in some respects in reaction to some of the ideas of Freud and his followers. The behavioral reaction that occurred first was away from the subjective mysteries of the mind of the psychodynamicists to what were thought to be the objective, observable realities of human action. However, the cognitive behaviorists have, in time, reacted against that imbalance to restore some mental element to the human equation. It is in the context of these two commonly used therapies that the reader is probably familiar with and that I now want to explore some of the major features of personal construct therapy.

The traditional assumptions by practitioners of *psychodynamic psychotherapy* about people, clients, and therapists hold that they have rich and powerful psychological phenomena, which occur at several different levels of awareness (Freud, 1925). These are the conscious, preconscious, and unconscious levels representing current awareness, potentially available awareness, and nonawareness. People's psyches are made up of primitive urges (id), the sensing, thinking, and judging functions (ego), and the internalized moral standards of society (super ego). Emotions and passions play an important part in this therapy. Anxiety from conflict between these aspects of their personalities and the demands of the worlds in which they live are handled by a range of defense mechanisms, such as denial and projection (Meltzer, 1978). Each of these mechanisms can be useful but its effect on their users, because each has its potential pitfalls, depends largely on how rigidly and blindly they use it. Therapy leading to insight into these processes is carried out using free associations, analysis of dreams, and interpretations of the transference of client to therapist. These concepts have been almost turned into structured objects, things to be manipulated, by some interpreters. However, some modern psychodynamic therapists are focusing now on the meanings of clients and therapists (Gill, 1976; Klein, 1976).

There are many different forms of *cognitive-behavioral therapy.* They include the self-efficacy approach of Bandura (1978), the cognitive restructuring of Beck (1976), and the rational-emotive therapy of Ellis (1984). All of these forms are based on the idea that the cognitions of clients are crucial to the changes in their problematic behavior that they want to achieve. It is the clients' cognitions that defeat them, so these cognitions need to be changed (Granvold, 1994). For Bandura, people interact with their world in such a way as to build up their self-efficacy or sense of personal power. It is, therefore, self-efficacy that moderates any therapeutic change. For Beck, Emery, and Greenberg (1985), clients develop nonadaptive meanings for their experiences, largely because they use inappropriate assumptions, faulty logic, and "automatic thoughts" which are self-derogatory. Such people do not recognize the differences between their cognitions about their worlds and the worlds in which they are living. Ellis, on the other hand, sees self-efficacy as irrelevant but is also concerned with the effects of irrational beliefs. These cognitive-behavioral approaches to therapy, perhaps because of their title, have been accused of ignoring emotion. Both Beck et al. and Ellis defended themselves against this criticism as inappropriate, but their accounts of therapy do indicate relatively little focus on powerful emotions and minimisation of negative emotions especially.

SOME IDEAS CHARACTERISTIC OF PERSONAL CONSTRUCT THERAPY

Some of the main ideas of personal construct therapy and the contrast of these ideas with those of other therapies are examined in the next section of this chapter. These ideas include the constructivist assumptions about people and psychotherapy, (which I discuss in greater detail in a later chapter of this book), and the views of both therapists and clients as construers, as well as their capacity for reconstruction.

Some General Ideas

Some important *ideas about the world* are considered first. Personal construct therapy differs from psychodynamic and cognitive-behavioral therapy in its assumptions about both the nature of our knowledge of reality and the concept of causation. Although these other therapeutic approaches assume reality to be directly accessible and stable personal construct therapy assumes it to be construed and variable (Mahoney & Lyndon, 1988). Furthermore, although these other approaches view causation as being demonstrated by chains of association, personal construct therapy considers it to involve the gradual refinement of people's representations of reality (Neimeyer, 1993).

Some important *ideas about people* are considered second. Trying to take a subjective as well as an objective view of people is central to personal construct therapy. Few psychodynamic therapists have also taken subjectivity to be central, although some, for instance Schafer (1983), do so. Adler (in Ansbacher & Ansbacher, 1956) also recognized early that the concepts of his theory were the creations of his own mind, designed to create meaning for his clients. More recently, a few psychodynamic therapists are beginning to consider a more constructivist view of therapy when they see their role as being able to discover jointly with their clients the meanings that are important to them (Schafer, 1983).

Two other general constructivist ideas remain for us to consider. One is the ability of people to behave "as if" their world were the "real" one. They can use their imagination to create events that may not even have happened and they can also use it to recreate past events. This capacity is a constructivist and not a psychodynamic one, although it can be seen in Adler's (Ansbacher & Ansbacher, 1956) psychodynamic therapy. The other idea is the ability of people to experience events at different levels of awareness. There are some events to which they will not have access or be able to describe. This is accepted by therapists like Freud (1925), as well as by Kelly (1955). Insight or self-understanding may be an important goal, then, for both of these therapists but in different ways. For example, for Freud, insight seemed to imply a full understanding of experienced events, whereas for Kelly, the constructivist, it is the effective use of one's own construct system to anticipate one's own actions. Neither of these ideas is compatible with the assumptions of cognitive-behavior therapy.

Some Ideas about Psychotherapy

Important *ideas about psychotherapy* are considered next. The main three constructivist ideas about psychotherapy are (a) therapy creates meaning, (b) therapy deals with change in meanings for clients, and (c) therapy takes place in a dialogue between therapists and clients (Kelly, 1955; Neimeyer, 1985). Therapy also can be seen as involving the telling of stories. Most psychodynamic therapists view therapy as creating new meanings for their clients and also for themselves; however, the type of meaning pursued is limited by therapists to that linked with psychodynamic concepts, compared with that in personal construct therapy in which meanings are largely defined by clients rather than therapists. The analyses of transference are examples of this. For psychodynamic therapists, it is the symbolic representation of people in their world that is said to lead to psychological problems. Some modern psychodynamicists are also now turning to the concept of narrative or story as an aid to the interpretation of meaning (Schafer, 1983), but they are wary of the power of the narrative as it can be told to convince falsely. Cognitive-behavioral therapists, on the other hand, are concerned with distorted cognitions and poor self-efficacy or little sense of competence. Problematic behavior is their focus for change. The concept of narrative can not be successfully applied to these therapies, either. Beck's automatic thoughts and Ellis's irrational beliefs lack the continuity and integration of stories.

Next are some ideas about *therapists as construers*. Probably the most important implication of the assumption that as a personal construct therapist I am a construer, or creator of personal meanings, is the requirement it makes of me to monitor my own construing and actions in therapy. This need has long been recognized in psychodynamic therapy by the concept of countertransference that has been developed to guard against the possibility of the subjective meanings of therapists holding power during therapy. In transference, the construing of important early relationships is transferred by clients from people in their everyday world to the relationship with the therapist. It is the interpretation of this process that forms the basis of effective therapy. In countertransference, however, it is the transfer of this construing of important early relationships in their own world to the relationship with the client that can distort the meaning of therapists. Countertransference is monitored carefully by psychodynamic therapists. However, the cognitive-behavioral approaches to therapy are not as reflexive as the psychodynamic approaches; that is, they do not apply as much to the therapist as the client. They do not use the idea of countertransference and the capacity of their therapists for self-monitoring can be limited by this.

Next are some ideas about *clients as construers*. When clients are assumed to be construers, it raises the question of how therapists assess the construing of those clients. In personal construct therapy, clients are seen as the expert on their own meanings. Most psychodynamic therapists (Freud, 1925) have, however, relied on guided accounts of their subjective worlds and free associations by their clients with interpretation of these productions by therapists for the assessment of their clients' construing. However, heuristic psychodynamicists, for example, do describe going through a process of mutual discovery of the meanings of their clients (Schafer, 1983). There is even a psychodynamic group that asserts that clients from childhood have beliefs about themselves that are self-defeating and that they come to therapy, planning, although unaware of this, to confirm them (Weiss, Sampson, & the Mount Zion Psychotherapy Research Group, 1986). Cognitive-behavioral therapists (Beck et al., 1985; Granvold, 1994) prefer in assessment to have objective observations of their clients' actions. Rational-emotive therapists (Beck, 1976; Ellis, 1984) are concerned with the assessment of what they see as the irrational beliefs of their clients, that is, meanings that are illogically inferred. Personal construct therapists do not take this objective view of their clients. They acknowledge their own subjective contribution to the therapeutic process.

Finally, *therapists and clients as reconstruers* are considered. Personal construct therapists and clients work together in therapy to find new meanings and tell new stories. The psychodynamic and cognitive-behavioral therapies tend rather to rely on the abilities of clients to reconstrue but do not expect so much reconstruction of their therapists. Psychodynamic therapists are concerned with how clients reconstrue, especially if they believe that their clients are planning to invalidate some of their most basic construing. Furthermore, if those psychodynamic therapists are working with clients to develop interpretations together, they may expect their own construing to change a little and not solely that of their clients (Casement, 1985). The cognitive-behavioral therapists, however, expect their clients but not themselves, to reconstrue. This is true of therapists who use cognitive restructuring, stress innoculation, and rational-emotive therapy.

SOME STRATEGIES CHARACTERISTIC OF PERSONAL CONSTRUCT THERAPY

The characteristic strategies of personal construct therapies that can be contrasted with those of two other groups of therapies described earlier include their selection of goals in therapy, the retelling of stories, and how this retelling is shared between therapists and clients. They also include some of the strategies they use in therapy (Mahoney & Gabriel, 1987).

The major *goals of personal construct therapy* for clients involve the achievement of greater awareness, the development of a range of alternative stories which they can apply to themselves, the making of some changes in what they do on the basis of these new stories, and, finally, the recognizing that there are choices to be made about the stories they tell about themselves. Neither psychodynamic nor cognitive-behavioral therapies share all of these constructivist goals. Psychodynamic therapists do see client awareness as important, whereas the cognitive-behavioral therapists do not. Neither of these therapies, however, focuses on alternatives and choices in the goals of their clients, as personal construct therapists do.

The *retelling of stories* plays a central role in this psychotherapy. In personal construct therapy, the stories told by clients are central to the therapeutic process. In psychodynamic and cognitive-behavioral therapy, stories are not so accepted. It can be argued, however, that these two therapies do provide, in their rival accounts of psychologically functioning, the alternative stories needed. Adler, the psychodynamic therapist, provided new stories about their power for his clients who continued to feel powerless even in adulthood and interpersonal narratives for clients he saw to be lacking in sociability. Rational-emotive therapy, too, helps its clients develop more rational beliefs about themselves and even a new life philosophy of rational debate. These therapists, however, come to therapy with specific stories with which they want their clients to leave, whereas personal construct therapists want their clients to emerge with stories that enable them to go on to serve as their own therapists.

Therapists and Clients Share the Retelling of Stories. Both therapists and clients make assumptions about psychotherapy that influence how it proceeds and have expectations about it that are also influential. As personal construct therapists come together with their clients, they share these assumptions and expectations as they share the process of retelling the stories of the therapy. As we retell our stories, I consider my clients to be as influential as I am. However, many therapists do not see their clients as cotherapists. Of the psychodynamic and cognitive-behavioral therapists that I am considering, few do so. This has been apparent in the way they write about their clients in therapy, as objective diagnosticians intent on minimizing their symptoms by training clients to accept their given prescriptions for care.

Therapists Come to Understand the Construing of their Clients. Personal construct therapists use a range of methods for understanding the construing of their clients, both initially and as therapy continues. Some of these assessment techniques are unique to personal construct therapy; others are not. The technique of listening to the constructs clients use as they talk is available. So, too, are techniques to assess the content of constructs (self-characterization), relationships between constructs (the Repertory Grid Technique), and to test how resistant constructs are to change (the ABC Technique). They are described in Chapter 10. More loose and imaginative techniques are also employed, such as listening to the stories of clients and much more rarely telling some of those of the therapist. These are shared with some psychodynamic therapists. The tighter and more constraining techniques are shared with some cognitive-behavioral therapists.

Therapists Helping Clients to Retell their Stories. Helping clients to retell their stories also involves therapists in using a range of therapeutic techniques. Analyzing their construing with them, asking them to act on the basis of that construing, and encouraging them to construe their own ability to construe are the primary constructivist strategies. However, many of those techniques that I report in this book as help in testing the predictive value of the construing of clients have been developed from the other theories of therapy with which I deal in this chapter. This is possible because the essence of personal construct therapy is testing and experimentation by both client and therapist. Free association and dream analysis can be useful contributions to personal construct therapy from the psychodynamic therapists, whereas cognitive restructuring, reframing, goal setting, prescriptions, homework, relaxation therapy, and assertiveness training can be useful contributions from the cognitive-behavioral therapists.

Although cognitive-behavioral therapists tend to be ahistorical and problem oriented, personal construct and psychodynamic therapists tend to be historical and process oriented. The same distinction between therapies also can be made with the notion of resistance on the part of the clients. Cognitive-behavioral therapists see it as a lack of motivation and failure of generalization in the learning process in clients, whereas personal construct and psychodynamic therapists see it as representing appropriate self-protection on their part. Although reconstruction can be said to take place in all four types of therapy, for the cognitive-behavioral therapists this process occurs through the monitoring of logic and reality testing by clients and therapists, whereas for personal construct and psychodynamic therapists it involves changes in the interpretations that clients and therapists make. A convenient summary of some of the differences and similarities between the ideas and strategies of personal construct therapy and those of the psychodynamic and cognitive-behavioral therapies is provided in Table 1.

Table 1.
Ideas and Strategies of Personal Construct Therapy Contrasted With Those of the Psychodynamic and Cognitive Behavioral Therapies

Ideas and Strategies	Personal Construct Therapy	Psychodynamic Therapy	Cognitive-Behavioral Therapy
About the World			
Knowledge of reality	Constructed representation	Reflection	Reflection
About People			
Perspective	Subjective	Objective	Objective
As if	Yes	No	No
Insight	Yes	Yes	No
About Therapy			
Meanings	Open	Limited	Limited
Stories	Useful	Dangerous	Inappropriate
Therapists as construers	Yes	Yes	No
Clients as construers	Yes	Yes	No
Joint reconstruction	Yes	To some extent	No
Therapy			
Goals	Awareness, alternative stories and choices	Awareness	Appropriate behavior
Storytelling	Important and chosen by clients	Less important and limited in content	Unimportant
Joint story telling	Yes	No	No
Methods for understanding clients	Wider range	Specific	Specific
Methods for helping clients	Any appropriate experiments	Specific	Specific
Focus	Historical, process	Historical, process	Ahistorical, problem

COMING TO UNDERSTAND PERSONAL CONSTRUCT THERAPY

This book provides a description of the change processes that occur in psychotherapy when it is viewed from a constructivist perspective. This perspective assumes both therapist and client to be active construers, making sense of themselves and one another. If you can use the basic counseling techniques of listening, reflection, and confrontation, you will be able to use this book to work effectively with clients. I begin the next section by identifying the ideas about people in general, which are basic to the constructivist approach, and follow that by considering those which are specifically about psychotherapy. In the next section, the construing of therapists and clients about themselves and psychotherapy is explored. Then the central role of reconstruing in psychotherapy is considered. In the fourth section, I deal in some depth with the reconstructive process, including the goals of personal construct therapy, the process of reconstruing, and the sharing of that reconstruing between therapist and client. In the fifth section of this book, I deal with some of the strategies of individual and group personal construct therapy.

Personal construct therapy provides a unique and challenging approach for therapists. I make sense of myself as a therapist in the same way that I make sense of my clients. Those constructivist ideas are applied to me just as they are applied to my clients, to provide accounts of our therapeutic goals, our beliefs about change and the importance of metaphor in our lives. We are also both seen as tellers of stories and as reconstruing our stories during psychotherapy. In order to make these points clear, I have described, in some detail, some examples of ongoing therapy with my own clients.

You now have choices to make about how you will read this book. I have written it in an order that seems appropriate to me, within the limits of my own construct system. You have your own system of constructs that directs your interests and reflects your experience of psychotherapy, in general, and personal construct therapy, in particular. If you are experienced and interested in theories of therapy, you may choose to go on to the next section of this book, to read more about the constructivist ideas. If your interests lie more in psychotherapeutic practice, you may choose to read next the middle sections on the construing and reconstruing of clients and therapists and the reconstructive process. You may also choose to continue by reading the three accounts of therapy cases in the Appendix at the end of the book, but if you do you will probably want to use the Glossary at the same time.

READINGS

Personal Construct Therapy

Bannister, D., & Fransella, F. (1985). *Inquiring man.* Chichester: Wiley.

Dalton, S., & Dunnett, G. (1993). *Living with personal construct psychology.* Chichester: Wiley.*

* Most useful readings.

Epting, F. (1984). *Personal construct counselling and therapy.* Chichester: Wiley.*
Kelly, G.A. (1955). *The psychology of personal constructs.* New York: Norton.*
Viney, L.L. (1993). The goals of reconstructive therapy: Reflections of a therapist. In G. Dunnett & L. Leitner (Eds.), *Critical issues in personal construct therapy.* Malabar, FL: Krieger.
Winter, D.A. (1990). Therapeutic alternatives for psychological disorder: Personal construct psychology investigations in a health service setting. In G.J. and R.A. Neimeyer (Eds.), *Advances in personal construct psychology.* Greenwich, CT: JAI.

Some Research Evaluating Personal Construct Therapy

Bannister, D., Adams-Webber, J.R., Penn, W.I., & Radley, A. (1975). Reversing the process of thought disorder: A serial validation experiment. *British Journal of Social and Clinical Psychology, 14,* 169–180.
Button, E. (1994). *Personal construct therapy for eating disorders.* Chichester: Wiley.
Evesham, M., & Fransella, F. (1985). Stuttering relapse: The effects of a combined speech and psychological reconstruction program. *British Journal of Disorders of Communication, 20,* 237–248.
Fransella, F. (1972). *Personal change and reconstruction: Research and treatment of stuttering.* London: Academic.
Karst, T.O., & Trexler, L.D. (1974). Initial study using fixed role and rational-emotive therapy in treating speaking anxiety. *Journal of Consulting and Clinical Psychology, 34,* 360–366.
McKain, T.L., Glass, C.R., Arnkoff, D.D., Sydnor-Greenberg, J.M., & Shea, C.A. (1988). Personal constructs and shyness: The relationship between Repertory Grid data and therapy outcome. *International Journal of Personal Construct Psychology, 1,* 151–167.
Neimeyer, R.A. (1993). An appraisal of constructivist psychotherapies. *Journal of Consulting and Clinical Psychology, 61,* 221–234.*
Sheehan, W.J. (1985). A personal construct study of depression. *British Journal of Medical Psychology, 72,* 197–209.
Viney, L.L. (1990). A constructivist model of psychological reactions to illness and injury. In G.J. & R.A. Neimeyer (Eds.), *Advances in personal construct psychology* (Vol. 1). Greenwich, CT: JAI.
Viney, L.L. (1993). Listening to what my clients say: Content analysis categories and scales. In G.J. Neimeyer (Ed.), *Casebook of constructivist assessment.* New York: Sage.
Viney, L.L. (1994). Sequences of emotional distress expressed by clients and acknowledged by therapists. *British Journal of Clinical Psychology, 33.* 469–481.
Viney, L.L., Benjamin, Y.N., & Preston, C.A. (1989). An evaluation of personal construct therapy for the elderly. *British Journal of Medical Psychology, 62,* 35–41.

Viney, L.L., Clarke, A.M., Bunn, T.A., & Benjamin, Y.N. (1985a). Crisis intervention counselling: An evaluation of long-term and short-term effects. *Journal of Counselling Psychology, 32,* 29–39.
Viney, L.L., Clarke, A.M., Bunn, T.A., & Benjamin, Y.N. (1985). The effects of a hospital-based counselling service on the physical recovery of surgical and medical patients. *General Hospital Psychiatry, 7,* 294–301.
Winter, D.A. (1992). *Personal construct psychology in clinical practice.* London: Routledge.

Two Other Psychotherapies

Bandura, A. (1978). The self system in reciprocal determinism. *American Psychologist, 33,* 344–358.
Beck, A.T. (1976). *Cognitive therapy and the emotional disorders.* New York: Meridian.
Beck, A.T., Emery, G., & Greenberg, R.L. (1985). *Anxiety disorders and phobias: A cognitive perspective.* New York: Basic Books.
Ellis, A. (1984). The essence of RET–1984. *Journal of Rational-Emotive Therapy, 2,* 19–26.
Freud, S. (1925). *The collected papers of Sigmund Freud.* London: Hogarth.
Gill, M. (1976). Metapsychologies not psychology. In M. Gill & P. Holzman (Eds.), Meta-psychology versus psychology: Psychoanalytic essays in memory of George S. Klein. *Psychological Issues, 9* (Mono. 36), 80–112.
Granvold, D.K. (1994). *Cognitive and behavioural treatment.* Monterey, CA: Brooks/Cole.
Klein, G. (1976). *Psychoanalytic theory.* New York: International Universities Press.
Meltzer, D. (1978). *The Kleinian development.* Strath Tay, Perthshire: Clunie Press.

Some Ideas Unique to Personal Construct Therapy

Ansbacher, H.L., & Ansbacher, R. (Eds.). (1956). *The individual psychology of Alfred Adler.* New York: Basic Books.
Casement, P. (1985). *On learning from the patient.* London: Tavistock.
Mahoney, M.J., & Lydon, W.J. (1988). Recent developments in cognitive approaches to counselling and psychotherapy. *The Counselling Psychologist, 16,* 190–234.*
Neimeyer, R.A. (1985). Personal constructs in clinical practice. In P.C. Kendall (Ed.), *Advances in cognitive-behavioural research and therapy.* New York: Academic.
Schafer, R. (1983). *The analytic attitude.* New York: Basic Books.
Weiss, J., Sampson, H., & The Mount Zion Psychotherapy Research Group. (1986). *The psychoanalytic process.* New York: Guilford.

Some Strategies Unique to Personal Construct Therapy

Mahoney, M.J., & Gabriel, T.J. (1987). Psychotherapy and the cognitive sciences: An evolving alliance. *Journal of Cognitive Psychotherapy, 1*, 39–59.

EXERCISES

1. Identify the major assumptions you make as a therapist about (a) your client and (b) yourself. Are these two sets of assumptions similar or different? How like those of personal construct therapy are they?
2. Apply the seven basic assumptions of personal construct therapy to some of your own thoughts, feelings, and actions. How are they useful?
3. Apply these assumptions to a client of yours. How are they useful?
4. Describe how some of the main ideas of personal construct therapists differ from those of psychodynamic therapists.
5. Describe how some of the main ideas of personal construct therapists differ from those of cognitive-behavioral therapists.

II

SOME IMPORTANT CONSTRUCTIVIST IDEAS

2

Constructivist Ideas About People

In this chapter, I deal with the main ideas about people that underlie personal construct therapy. They include a focus on our subjectivity, our meanings, how we create those meanings, and exercise our intentions and purposes. Other relevant constructivist ideas deal with the flexibility of our construing, the different levels of our awareness, the relation between construing and emotion, the uniqueness of the individual construing of each of us, and our shared meanings, as well as some of the ideas of social constructionism. Social constructionism and personal construct theory are both based on these constructivist assumptions.

Throughout this book my discussion of the ideas underlying personal construct therapy are illustrated by accounts of therapy in which I have been involved as the therapist. The clients described have all been referred to my university-based clinic and their identities have been disguised so as to maintain my contracts of confidentiality with them. The two clients whose therapies are discussed in this and the next section of the book are Christine and Frank. Christine, at 29 years of age, reported much anxiety and depression to her physician, who, finding her to be physically healthy, referred her to my clinic. She was working to support her husband financially, he being a full-time graduate student. Frank, at 45 years of age, was referred by the courts after being charged with damage to property. The anger underlying this behavior was sometimes stimulated by alcohol, but not always. He was living alone, with occasional part-time work to supplement his unemployment benefit. He was a diabetic needing a daily dose of insulin which he, himself, injected. He also had a diabetes-related diet, to which he only sometimes kept faithful. The stories of the struggles of these two people to reconstrue, and mine as their therapist to help them reconstrue, will show the implications of these ideas for what is done in therapy.

THE MAJOR CONSTRUCTIVIST IDEAS ABOUT PEOPLE

Personal Meanings

Whether to take a *subjective or an objective perspective* on people has long been debated by psychotherapists. Should I try to understand others from an internal and personal or an external and less personal frame of reference? Many of my therapist colleagues take the latter perspective. However, for constructivists, the subjective frame of reference is of great importance (Kelly, 1955, chap. 2). They consider all knowledge to be personal knowledge (Polanyi & Prosch, 1975; Popper, 1989). That is not to say that there is no objective reality, but that people can only come close to knowing it by creating better subjective accounts of it. This idea could lead to an extreme form of relativism in which all accounts of people as being equally tenable with no criteria by which to evaluate their relative merits. Careful study of the internal consistency of peoples' construing of their world can help to guard against this problem (May, 1964). So can checking their accounts with those of other people. The philosophy of phenomenology helps, too, with its concern that people be aware of assumptions and reflect with rigor when they develop their accounts of clients (Jennings, 1986; Spinelli, 1989). When Christine and Frank arrived for their first therapy sessions, as their therapist I began by trying to understand their view of what was happening to them. I also reflected on my own assumptions about the experiences of people, in general, and those of Christine and Frank, in particular.

There is, too, a form of constructivism that maintains not only that knowledge is subjectively created, but also that it is created through interaction between people. This is social constructionism (Gergen, 1985). Psychologies that are based on this idea provide accounts of people that are less impersonal and out of context than many current psychologies do. They also transcend the traditional conflict between the taking of subjective and objective viewpoints. In terms of therapy, this means that therapists move, as quickly as the client and they are able, toward building some shared constructs. Their progress is influenced by how each of them is functioning. In Christine's first session, this was achieved quite quickly as we discussed the reasons for her referral. We soon had a shared picture of the events, including a suicide bid which had led to it. With Frank this was not achieved for many sessions, partly because Frank's construing of the events which led to his referral was, to say the least, confused. My initial construing of him was tinged with this confusion but I was able to reflect on this confusion as it seemed likely to be similar to the experience of other people meeting with Frank. My understanding of his confusion enabled me to accept it as part of my experience of our early therapeutic interaction and wait to see what else I would experience with him.

The constructivist acceptance of the important role of subjectivity in any account of people is closely linked with an acceptance of *meaning* as crucial to constructivist psychologies (Bannister & Fransella, 1986; Mair, 1989). People try to make sense of what happens to them. Therefore, any understanding of people that forms the basis of a personal construct therapy must view both therapists and clients as searching for meaning. The methods for the understanding of subjective meanings coming from phenomenology have been most effective. As far as the phenomenological reflection and examination of constructs to which I have referred, there is the technique of description (Keen, 1972). I find that phenomenological description requires of me considerable self-understanding and self-control. With both Christine and Frank, I tried to arrive at their phenomenological description of the events that led to their referrals, that is, to the meanings of those events for each of them. Christine was able to make sense of her attempt to commit suicide, in terms of what she perceived to be her loneliness and alienation from others: "I thought: Nobody cares about me; I might as well end it all." Frank took much longer to achieve a personal meaning for his property damage, of which more emerges as we follow his therapy further. I must wonder, of course, how much this was due to my own construing. It is certainly easier for me to imagine myself depressed than it is to imagine myself breaking someone else's window. It was therefore particularly important in my work with Frank that I clearly articulate my meanings for the events of our therapy and use them to work therapeutically with him.

Meaning is Created. Meaning is not thrust on people. They actively impose meaning on their experiences; their experiences do not impose it on them (Mahoney, 1988). Meaning is created by the act of construing. Clients and therapists create meanings. As even infants meet with new experiences, it seems likely that they create personally meaningful constructs for them. Yet, it is only when they are later able to talk to others that they can share these meanings. These constructs are often about self (Epting & Amerikaner, 1980). Many of these personal meanings serve to maintain a sense of the integrity of how self is experienced and the continuity of that experience over time. Of course, if people can create their own meanings, they can also change them (Guidano & Liotto, 1985; Mahoney & Freeman, 1985). Such reconstruing is the essence of psychotherapy.

When clients come to psychotherapy for the first time, they need to make sense of their new experiences, using either meanings which they have employed effectively with other events or new meanings which they have created. As a therapist, I try to understand those meanings. Christine's response to my question about how she saw my role in our work together during our first session was slow to come but instructive. She saw me initially as "pointing out what I'm doing wrong," which proved to be a construct much in evidence in relation to her mother. She did not see me as like her boss, however, whom she saw as supportive. This view of me was to change later. Frank had great difficulty in articulating any meaning for me as his therapist and eventually settled for a while on seeing me like "a doctor, who would make sure everything is okay."

How is Meaning Construed? How do I make sense of my clients' meanings? Some literary theorists maintain that the single elements of a story only have meaning as part of the whole story (Eagleton, 1983). It may follow that people's meanings for their experienced events can only be understood in the context of their lives (Hermans, Kemper, & Van Loon, 1992; Keating & Rosen, 1991; Markova, 1987). Even if this is so, there is still the question of whether meaning is arrived at through comparisons resulting from similarities or differences (Burr & Butt, 1992). Frank appeared to use only similarities in his early attempts to construe me as his therapist. However, Christine used both similar and different points of comparison. So did I, as I tried to make their comments meaningful in the light of my own constructs. I particularly compared what I heard them say, and what I saw of their actions when making statements, with earlier clients who had reported similarly to or differently from them. This helped me to begin to understand their meanings better.

Constructivists take the view that both types of comparison are necessary (R.A. Neimeyer, 1995). Indeed, such comparisons are seen as resulting in constructs that are bipolar (Holland, 1970; Kelly, 1969). Bipolar constructs provide paths between which clients can choose. All clients, then, whether they are aware of it or not, have choices they can make. For example, initially, Christine was construing herself using a construct with the twin poles of fearful and confident. She wished to be confident but saw herself as fearful, whereas she saw me as confident. Each construct is useful in predicting only a limited range of events. People test them continually in their day-to-day interactions.

When their predictions are confirmed, validation is said to have occured. When their predictions are not confirmed, it is invalidation that occurs. People develop systems of constructs that can influence or be influenced by one another. Superordinate constructs influence, whereas subordinate ones are influenced. How people use their constructs will be governed in part by this superordinacy. It is necessary, then, for us to understand something of the construct system and the relations of these constructs of our clients before our therapy can be effective.

Imagination and Anticipation

Another major idea is that people are able to *act as if their view of the world were real* when that may not be the case (Kelly, 1964; Vaihinger, 1911).

They can use their imaginations to both represent and experiment with events. Clients and therapists act in response to their own construing rather than to events as such. Constructivists are rigorous relativists; that is, we accept that a number of accounts of events will be available but evaluate them carefully (Rychlak, 1982; Viney, 1987). I therefore recognize the subjectively created quality of my account of my clients but continually test its usefulness as a predictor. For those clients, it is important to be able to proceed as if in order to test the predictive value of their construing. For me as a therapist, it is equally important for my part in the designing of such tests.

The use of imagination is, then, very important to personal construct therapy. Neither Christine nor Frank found this task easy in their first session. I tried to help Christine, for example, to test the resistance of her negative construing of herself to change. Her as-if world was one of: "Nothing will turn out right for me." This represented a view of herself that seemed in conflict, to me, with evidence of her good academic performance at school. When I gently confronted her with this, she minimized the evidence that I used: "Oh, that was nothing. I had no real competition. When I went on to university I found out what real competition was like."

People have *goals* that they intend to achieve (Rychlak, 1968, 1981; Viney, 1992). They use predictions, to plan for these projects. In other words, effective anticipation is important to them (Neimeyer, 1995). My clients and I predict what makes most sense to us; given the content and structure of our construct systems we have a sense of the future and can be said to have purpose. What this means for personal construct therapy is that both my clients and I are seen as coming to it with goals or purposes to be achieved. As a therapist, I try to articulate such goals as clearly and as quickly as possible. For my clients, however, clear articulation may be longer in coming. Frank could find no answer to my enquiry about what he wanted from therapy. His main response to the question was confused anger: "It's fucking-well nothing to do with me. I was sent here. I don't really. . . ." I needed several sessions with Frank before I could state clearly the projects I thought we could work toward in relation to that anger. I think that my own goal in therapy with him was about seeing myself as an effective therapist, and I was far from realization at this stage. However, I had seen myself as an effective therapist with earlier clients so I could therefore wait longer with some confidence to see what happened with Frank.

OTHER IDEAS ABOUT PEOPLE

In this introduction to a constructivist psychology, I focused so far on its most important ideas. Their implications for personal construct therapy include that both my clients should understand our own subjectivity, meaning, created meaning, our construction of meaning, our as-if worlds, and our goals. Now I turn to some other constructivist ideas. They have to do with the flexibility of our construing, the different levels of our awareness, and the close relation between our construing and our emotion. Both the uniqueness of individual meanings and the role of shared meanings together with some further implications of social constructionism are considered.

Flexibility of Construing, Levels of Awareness and Emotions

The *flexibility* of people as they construe events is often remarkable (Mahoney, 1988). My clients and I have the ability to construe loosely and to construe tightly. When we construe loosely many alternative predictions are possible; however, when we construe tightly only specific unvarying predictions are made. Frank showed loose construing when he spoke of "not knowing how the therapy-thing might turn out." However, he showed tight construing when he added, thinking of his unemployment benefit: "But I can't come on Tuesdays because that is dole day." People differ in how flexible their construing is. It depends, as well as on their ability to move between tight and loose construing, on the permeability of their constructs. A permeable construct can be used to account for new events; an impermeable one cannot. Christine showed an impermeable construct at work when she said of her job as a secretary: "Even if I could see that I did good work at school, I can't see that it applies to me as I am now." My construing was, I believe, permeable, when initially as Frank's therapist I said to myself: "I don't understand him fully now; but I have not understood new clients often in the past but have come to understand them, so maybe I will come to understand Frank too."

Several *levels of awareness* are considered possible in this approach. All experienced events are assumed by constructivists to be potentially accessible to awareness. Insight, then, is an important goal for both clients and therapists (Kelly, 1955, chap. 2). Insight can be understood as the effective use of one's own construct system to anticipate one's own actions. Different levels of awareness are possible (Kelly, 1955; Rychlak, 1983). Those levels have much to do with whether constructs are preverbal or verbal. In other words, constructs at low levels of awareness may be identified by their failure to be communicated verbally or their existence outside the range of one's most important constructs. Preverbal constructs have often been originally found when we were young children, before we developed the power of speech. As an example of preverbal construing, I had a vague awareness of an understanding of Frank's world as he talked with me that I could not put into words until much later in our relationship. Low levels of awareness may also be apparent because one pole of the entire construct may not be accessible or the entire construct may have been suspended. Later in therapy with Christine, she proved to have dropped a construct of "efficient versus inefficient," although it had been actively used by her for construing events earlier in her life. This selective lack of awareness later appeared to have been in response to the stress of demands for impossible amounts of work from her in her job, which she mistook for her inefficient construct pole.

I also want to make two other comments on the concept of awareness. Insight implies not only "I know," but also "I know that I know." Reflection is an integral component of awareness. The other relevant comment concerns low levels of awareness again and stems from acceptance of the as-if assumption. If there are many alternative views of events, then no one view is the correct one. There is mine, and yours, and theirs. Lack of awareness of experience can only be construed from an external rather than internal perspective. For example, when I initially construed Frank as angry, he did not seem to be aware of this feeling. It was only by using my own construct system in conjunction with his that it became possible for me to write in my early therapy notes: "Frank seems unaware of his anger, which I am seeing in his swearing and sometimes violent movements." My construing that he was angry was made on the basis of a construct that was mainly built on my experiences of other, similar people.

The *relation between construing and emotion* in this approach is a very close one. Construing and emotion have been separated by Anglo Saxon philosophers and psychologists for centuries. Some constructivists, too, have tended to follow this path. Personal construct theory has made one of the most successful attempts to integrate them into one account of how people function (Fransella & Dalton, 1990). This theory is concerned with changes: changes in construing and changes in actions. People are seen by it as in the process of continual transition. Yet, change brings the risk of invalidation of construing when predictions are not confirmed. The distressing emotions arise when construing is not validated and constructs are in conflict (Fransella & Dalton, 1990). Emotion-based interpretations and anticipations are active to a greater or lesser extent at all times, presetting construct systems and directing attention (Miall, 1989). Two examples will suffice: anger and anxiety. First, a constructivist account of anger is provided. Anger occurs when people whose constructs are invalidated continue to try to get validation of those constructs (McCoy, 1980). During our early sessions, Frank would suddenly break off our fruitful negotiations to vacillate between verbal abuse and uncooperative sulking. It eventually proved that he held a construct that viewed all women as caregivers. My approach to him was more that of a constructive collaborator than a caregiver, yet he was still trying to get validation for his own construing of me. It took several sessions to bring this to a higher level of awareness for us both.

The second example of an emotion understood in terms of construing is anxiety. Anxiety is experienced by people when they recognize that the event they are construing is beyond the range of their construct (McCoy, 1980). Each construct can be appropriately applied to sets of events but some events must be beyond the range of some constructs. The total construct system, of course, has a wider range of events of which it makes sense. Christine in her initial session expressed some anxiety about being in therapy. She was tense and defensive and construed therapy as "only for weak people." Because she did not construe herself as weak, this meant that her constructs relating to therapy did not range as far as her own action of coming to therapy. Naturally, she was anxious. I explored with her the possibility of viewing coming to therapy as a strong and courageous act; however, several sessions went by before she was able to construe herself in that way. Of course, as a therapist I can also experience anxiety when some therapy events are beyond the range of my constructs. One of the advantages of being an experienced therapist is that as my experiences build up, the more extensive and elaborate the parts of my construct systems dealing with therapy, and so the less anxiety I experience. This anxiety was not so much with Christine, whom I felt I understood, as for Frank, whose moves from verbal to physical abuse, which were quite common for him, I was still working on being able to predict.

People as Unique and as Sharers

Uniqueness is important to the constructivist approach to people in at least two ways. The first of these is that people structure their worlds uniquely (Bannister & Fransella, 1986). The construct systems of both therapists and clients are the unique products of their interactions with their worlds. My own constructs about therapy, for example, are a unique blend of concepts and techniques from psychoanalytic, cognitive-behavioral, and personal construct therapy and from my experiences as both client and therapist. Yet, they are also unique from an internal perspective. Each of us, when construing ourselves, sees him- or herself as unique (Salmon, 1980). Both Christine and Frank expressed strongly the uniqueness they experienced, especially in relation to the problems which had brought them to therapy. Christine, for example, said frequently: "No-one knows how bad I feel. No one else could feel like that." As her therapist, I was also aware of at least the potential for uniqueness of her construct systems; I pressed myself to attend primarily to her individual construing, rather than slip into assuming its similarity to that of other clients who had spoken and acted as she had.

Meanings are shared. Although uniqueness is important to the constructivist approach, that approach also takes the view that meanings can be shared (Mair, 1990). If meanings could not be shared, communication, the basis of psychotherapy, would not be possible. Some constructivists go so far as to claim that people's construing is meaningful only if it is shared. This is the criterion that has been accepted by many scientists as showing whether their construings are meaningful (Popper, 1989). Others see the role of shared meanings as rather different. For personal construct therapists, if two people construe the same event in similar ways, they are said to have similar psychological processes. They may belong to the same culture. In therapy, clients and therapists construe in ways that are both similar and different. I shared many meanings with Christine and Frank, largely because we were all members of an English-speaking culture. We shared more meanings, too, because for all of us that culture was the same. However, there were also many meanings of theirs that I did not share, especially about the problems which brought them to therapy. In that area, some of my construing was drawn from a different culture of which this book is a part, the culture of the psychotherapist.

Some *constructs from social constructionism* are relevant to personal construct psychology. There is a type of constructivist approach called social constructionism that goes beyond shared individual meaning to the notion that all meanings are socially created (Gergen, 1985). It is based on the work of the sociologist Alfred Schütz (1972). Schütz explored the implications of constructivist assumptions for interpersonal relationships, groups, and cultures, whereas George Kelly pursued them primarily with individuals. Yet, psychotherapy involves interpersonal relationships; it takes place within a cultural context. These ideas are very important, then, to a constructivist approach to therapy.

All construing of events is said to be a socially creative act. All knowledge, then, is socially construed. All knowledge is gained through communal interchange; although it may not be universally shared, it is socially created. The concept of social construction has been usefully applied, for example, to the problem of unemployment. Unemployment is socially construed in Western cultures as demeaning. Yet, because we construed that demeaning role for the unemployed, we can reconstrue it and set up new roles for them. Our personal meanings for unemployment have somehow almost become objective realities. There is a danger of this inappropriate objectification of the subjective occuring with psychotherapy, in the pressures to write and do research about it from a purely external viewpoint. The ideas of social constructionism are now being applied to psychotherapy (McNamee & Gergen, 1992).

THE MAJOR CONSTRUCTIVIST IDEAS ABOUT PEOPLE

Psychotherapy must however be, in part, at least a personal experience seen from an internal viewpoint and shared from another internal viewpoint; it is about this that I write. In the next chapter, I examine some of the important ideas of this approach about psychotherapy.

READINGS

Major Constructivist Ideas About People

Bannister, D., & Fransella, F. (1986). *Inquiring man.* Beckenham: Croom Helm.

Gergen, K.J. (1985). The social constructionist movement in modern psychology. *American Psychologist, 40,* 266–275.

Jennings, J.L. (1986). Husserl revisited: The forgotten distinction between psychology and phenomenology. *American Psychologist, 41,* 1231–1240.

Keen, E. (1972). *Psychology and the new consciousness.* Monterey, CA: Brooks/Cole.

Kelly, G.A. (1955). *The psychology of personal constructs*. New York: Norton.*
Mair, J.M.M. (1989). *Between psychology and psychotherapy: A poetry of experience*. London: Routledge.
May, R. (1964). On the phenomenological bases of psychotherapy. *Review of Existensial Psychology and Psychiatry, 4,* 22–36.
Neimeyer, R.A. (1995). Constructivist psychotherapies: Features foundation and future directions. R. In R.A. Neimeyer & M.J. Mahoney (Eds.), *Constructivism in psychotherapy*. Washington, DC: American Psychological Association.
Polanyi, M., & Prosch, H. (1975). *Meaning*. Chicago: University of Chicago Press.
Popper, K.R. (1989). *The logic of scientific discovery*. New York: Basic Books.
Spinelli, L. (1989). *The interpreted world*. London: Sage.

Other Ideas About People

Burr, V.S., & Butt, T. (1992). *Invitation to personal construct psychology*. London: Shurr.
Eagleton T. (1983). *Literary theory*. Minneapolis: University of Minneapolis Press.
Epting, F., & Amerikaner, M. (1980). Optimal functioning: A personal construct approach. In A.W. Landfield & L.M. Leitner (Eds.), *Personal construct psychology: Psychotherapy and personality*. New York: Wiley.
Fransella, F., & Dalton, P. (1990). *Personal construct counselling in action*. London: Sage.
Guidano, V.F., & Liotto, G. (1985). A constructivist foundation for cognitive therapy. In M.J. Mahoney & A. Freeman (Eds.), *Cognition and psychotherapy*. New York: Plenum.
Hermans, H.J.M., Kempen, H.J.G., & Van Loon, R.J.P. (1992). The dialogical self: Beyond individualism and rationalism. *American Psychologist, 47,* 23–32.
Holland, R. (1970). George Kelly: Constructive innocent and reluctant existensialist. In D. Bannister (Ed.), *Perspectives in personal construct theory*. London: Academic.*
Keating, D.P., & Rosen, H. (1991). *Constructivist perspectives on developmental psychopathology and atypical development*. Hillsdale, NJ: Erlbaum.
Kelly, G.A. (1964). The language of hypothesis: Man's psychological instrument. *Journal of Individual Psychology, 20,* 137–152.*
Kelly, G.A. (1969). Epilogue: Don Juan. In B. Maher (Ed.), *Clinical psychology and personality*. New York: Wiley.
Lincoln, Y.S. (1990). The working of a constructivist: A remembrance of transformations past. In E.G. Guba (Ed.), *The paradigm dialogue*. London: Sage.

---

* Most useful readings.

Mahoney, M.J. (1988). Constructivist metatheory: I. Basic features and historical foundations. *International Journal of Personal Construct Psychology, 1,* 1–36.*

Mahoney, M.J., & Freeman, A. (Eds.). (1985). *Cognition and psychotherapy.* New York: Plenum.

Mair, J.M.M. (1990). Telling psychological tales. *International Journal of Personal Construct Psychology, 3,* 1–22.

Markova, I. (1987). *Paradigms, thought and language.* Chichester: Wiley.

Mc Coy, M. (1980). Positive and negative emotion: A personal construct theory interpretation. In H. Bonarius, R.S. Holland, & S. Rosenberg (Eds.), *Recent advances in the theory and practice of personal construct psychology.* London: Macmillan.*

McNamee, S., & Gergen, K.J. (Eds.). (1992). *Therapy as social construction.* London: Sage.

Miall, D.S. (1989). Anticipating the self: Towards a personal construct construct model of emotion. *International Journal of Personal Construct Psychology, 2,* 185–198.

Neimeyer, G.J., & Neimeyer, R.A. (1993). Defining the boundaries of constructivist assessment. In G.J. Neimeyer (Ed.), *Constructivist assessment.* New York: Sage.

Rychlak, J.F. (1968). *A philosophy of science of personality.* Boston: Houghton Mifflin.

Rychlak, J.F. (1981). *Introduction to personality and psychotherapy.* Boston: Houghton Mifflin.

Rychlak, J.F. (1982). Some therapeutic implications of logical phenomenology. *Psychotherapy, 19,* 259–265.

Rychlak, J.F. (1983). Exclusivity in psychological specialization: A conceptual or practical problem? *Journal of Social & Clinical Psychology, 1,* 185–192.

Salmon, P. (1980). *Coming to know.* London: Routledge & Kegan Paul.

Schütz, A. (1972). *Phenomenology of the social world.* Portsmouth, NH.: Heineman.

Vaihinger, H. (1911). *The philosophy of as if.* Berlin: Reuter & Reuter.

Viney, L.L. (1987). *Interpreting the interpreters: Strategies for a science of construing people.* Malabar, FL: Krieger.

Viney, L.L. (1992). Can we see ourselves changing? Toward a constructivist model of adult psychosocial development. *Human Development, 36,* 65–75.

EXERCISES

1. Remember some recent experiences of a situation that was new to you and show how you made it meaningful for yourself.
2. Identify both poles of a bipolar construct that a client of yours is

using to make sense of the world. What choices do these poles offer him or her?

3. Identify a preverbal construct used by a client of yours. How is it influencing how he or she acts?
4. When did you recently feel angry? Identify the actions you used to try to secure validation for your invalidated construing.
5. When did you recently feel anxious? Describe the events that were beyond the range of your construct system that led to that anxiety.

3

Constructivist Ideas About Psychotherapy

The important constructivist ideas specific to psychotherapy that I have chosen to deal with are: (a) defining therapy as creating meaning and as providing the opportunity for both participants to develop new meanings about themselves and their worlds, (b) the main area of change in therapy is assumed to be meanings related to oneself and one's world, (c) therapy is seen as occurring through a dialogue between client and therapist who share a focus through the meeting of their construct systems, and (d) therapy is viewed as storytelling.

PSYCHOTHERAPY CREATES MEANING

Psychotherapy is about meaning (Bannister, 1975; Hobson, 1985; Viney, 1981). It focuses on the meanings of therapists and those of their clients (Epting, 1981). It even involves the creation of new meanings as they share meanings (Barton, 1974). The clients' meanings are often seen as the focus of therapy, although therapists' meanings are just as important to therapy. Clients' communication of their meanings also sometimes seem to have become distorted and as needing psychotherapy to right that distortion. This was probably so for both Christine, and Frank, when they began therapy. Their expression of some of their most fundamental construing was permeated by the dominating emotions they were experiencing. For Christine, this emotion was depressive in tone; for Frank, it was angry. In the course of therapy, they both needed to create new meanings out of their internal chaos.

CHANGE IN THE MEANING OF SELF

The main area of change in psychotherapy is I, me, and mine in the context of my world (Goldfried, 1982). Or, rather, to constructivists, it is the client's experience of him- or herself and the people of the client's world that is the focus of change (Guidano, 1991). Although I apply this construct readily to my clients, I must also be careful to apply it to myself as a therapist (Guidano & Liotto, 1985). I deal with my clients, however, for the moment. In therapy, they learn about themselves. They are developing knowledge about themselves in relation to others in their worlds. They are learning, more specifically, about their own uniqueness and individuality and their own intactness and continuity as an experiencing person. They also come to reconstrue others by using the construing they have recently developed for themselves (Katakis, 1989). Eventually they come to acknowledge their own abilities as construers or creators of meaning (Neimeyer & Neimeyer, 1993).

Frank and Christine again serve as examples. Frank proved to have a very weak sense of the continuity of his own experience. Many people in their midlife have detached from their childhood experiences but they have a sense of continuity that goes back some 10 or 20 years. Perhaps his obvious unhappiness at school and home had something to do with this. Frank said of all these periods of his life: "It's as if they happened to someone else." He needed to find his own role as the integrator of these experiences. Christine, on the other hand, was concerned to develop knowledge about her depressed view of herself and her world over which she felt very little power. She needed to acknowledge that she, herself, had created her depressive construing and so was able to create a more satisfying construing of herself and events.

PSYCHOTHERAPY AS CONSTRUCTIVE DIALOGUE

Psychotherapy is a dialogue between clients and therapists in which meanings are developed. That has been the meaning of dialogue almost 2,500 years since Plato and Aristotle (Entralgo, 1970). It is a constructive dialogue in that it involves the interaction of two construct systems (Winter, 1992). It follows from this assumption that therapists should make sense of themselves using the same meanings that they apply to their clients (Kelly, 1955, chap. 3 & 10). This view of therapy as dialogue implies that clients and therapists will both change as they communicate with each other. If the interview of psychological research can be analyzed as dialogue, as it has been, then the psychotherapy interview can also be viewed in that way. The techniques of psychotherapy then become those that start and maintain such dialogue.

Dialogues between my construct system and those of Christine and Frank were initiated in the first sessions of therapy. For example, my construing of people with psychological problems, based on both my personal and professional experiences, at the time I met with Christine, was that they may have very polarized construing of at least one parent. I therefore predicted that she would use only one pole of at least one of her bipolar construct, as she talked about her parents, and not move easily between the two. Our dialogue ran as follows:

Linda:	How about your parents? Do you have strong feelings about either of them?
Christine:	No, well . . . to be honest . . . Mum is pretty difficult, she has always been very critical of me. Even at school when I tried to please her by getting her a nice birthday present or something, she could always see something wrong with it.
Linda:	Can you tell me about a particular time when this happened?
Christine:	Oh, I put a lot of effort into getting her a book that I thought she wanted for her birthday and she said it cost too much [sigh].
Linda:	And you feel sad and frustrated by that.
Christine:	Yes, I do still. And angry . . .

Therapy can be seen as a dialogue between two views of how meanings are created, that of the client and of the therapist. When clients and therapists come to the dialogue of psychotherapy, they bring with them construing about how certain important aspects of therapy will proceed (Joyce-Moniz, 1985). Personal construct therapy focuses on the clients' self and world, so both clients and therapists bring interpretations and predictions to therapy (Kenny, 1987). For me, part of what is brought is my private and personal construing, but some of the remainder is publicly shared construing in the form of psychological theories about how people function. More of the remainder is likely to be shared construing about how psychological change occurs (Hayhow & Levy, 1989).

As I met with Frank initially, I had a stream of construing about him that was fed by theories of psychotherapy:

Linda:	(How does Frank see himself? Does he hold so called "irrational" ideas about himself, as the ra-

tional-emotive therapists suggest, or is his anger a reaction to deep intrapsychic conflicts?)

An important part of the rest of the publicly shared construing in therapy is about how meanings are developed. Psychologists are calling for more attention to the study of the epistemologies or theories of meaning (Lamiell, 1987). They have examined the epistemologies of therapists and found that they fall into three main types (Schacht & Black, 1985). The first of these is empiricism, in which the value of the construing of clients is tested against the relevant objective observations, although observations which are relevant may be difficult to find in therapy. The second is rationalism, with a criterion of logical consistency for construing. This, again, does not appear to be appropriate for all people in all situations. The third type of therapist epistemology is metaphorism, in which the value of construing is tested against the criterion of how individual meanings fit into wider meaning structures. Needless to say, the third is the epistemology closest to my heart. However, clients and therapists come to the therapeutic dialogue with different epistemologies, so some negotiation of how meaning is construed in therapy is necessary. For example, Christine initially saw our creation of meaning as my responsibility, whereas I saw it as our joint responsibility:

Christine: You know so much more about people with problems than I do.

Linda: I don't know more about you, though. I can supply some ideas for us to work with, but you are the one who is the expert on you and what you are experiencing.

Christine: I suppose . . . (doubtfully); but I don't know what to do about myself.

PSYCHOTHERAPY AS STORYTELLING

I now move from these constructivist assumptions about psychotherapy to suggest that construing can be seen as storytelling. In other words, I use the epistemology of metaphorism. Furthermore, construing may be described as resulting in coherent and useful stories when it meets certain criteria. Such stories play a role in the lives of all of us: clients and therapists. Theories of therapy are stories and therapy is an exchange of stories between clients and therapists. Psychotherapy may then be construed as storytelling.

Constructing stories can be important to therapy. Construing, similarly, may be seen as narrative (Britton & Pellegrini, 1990). The concept of narrative is used to refer to the plot of a succession of incidents, or story. This idea of story provides a focus on the meanings of therapists and clients that is broader than the content of a single construct, which could oversimplify, but narrower than a whole construct system, which could be too complex. It shows one or more constructs in use for construing a number of events concerning self and others. Stories seem more likely to be used when people act and make choices. People even think and feel in terms of stories (Nash, 1990). A growing number of psychologists would like to see the use of this metaphor in our construing of people in general and not only in psychotherapy (Sarbin, 1986).

But what is a story? A story provides a sequence of meanings, or constructs, that come together to form a single theme of a higher order (Kurtzman, 1987). Stories integrate different elements of experience to achieve that overriding whole and that whole has a different meaning from its separate parts. Stories are internally cohesive and consistent (Carr, 1985). There are meaningful relations between the parts of stories, each of which has a different meaning. These relations form a comprehensive whole, which may be loosely or tightly integrated. A story also has a time dimension. The integration of constructs and events I have referred to takes place over time to provide continuity, even though the storyteller may introduce the parts of the story nonsequentially. When a story meets these criteria, it is likely to have an impact on storyteller and listener alike.

Stories play many roles in peoples' lives (Hoshmand, 1993). For example, those people who can maintain a personal story in the face of life's changes are likely to maintain a sense of the continuity and coherence of themselves (Cohler, 1982). Each individual life is a story, as can be seen from the reminiscences of the elderly (Viney, 1993). Crisis is a way of making a story out of the lack of sense of some people's chaotic lives. Self and world is always the context of the story (Dennett, 1983). Self is the center around which people organize their stories. When people are unable to tell their stories, their construing of themselves becomes very limited in scope. Therapists and clients have different stories about the psychotherapy that occurs and so would any observer of their interaction. This means that psychotherapy research carried out with this constructivist perspective should include stories of therapy from all three of these perspectives.

Theories of therapy may be seen as as stories. Personal construct therapy has been described as a story (Mair, 1989). Yet, it is not the only theory of psychotherapy to be so described. All theories of therapy, as expressed by their therapists during psychotherapy, provide alternative stories for clients by which to live their lives and organize their therapeutic changes (Murphy & Medin, 1985). Theories of therapy provide ways to see connections between meanings. This integration is the essence of integrative narrative. I find that the story of therapy that develops during psychotherapy is largely mine as therapist but that it is modified to some extent to fit with the story of my client.

Psychotherapy is storytelling. When psychotherapy is considered to be discourse, it is a dialogue shaped by the asking and answering of questions. Psychotherapy, in other words, is the joint product of the stories that clients and therapists tell. Yet, they have the ability to organize stories from separate events (Viney, 1988). Psychotherapy goes beyond these stories to create new stories jointly between therapists and clients (Winter, 1988). Analysis of such stories could provide some answers to the criticisms of psychotherapy process research. However, my current concern is with the therapeutic meaning of these stories. Did Christine have a story to share with me, her therapist?

She was concerned to account for her attempt at suicide and this was the story she told.

Christine: I don't know what made me do it, or even what led up to it. Let me think. I was very busy at work, I remember. The pressure was really on at the end of the tax year; and Peter was finishing his thesis, so he didn't have much time for me. I hadn't spoken to Mum and Dad for months, so . . . No, I don't know what set me off like that.

As her therapist, with my own complementary stories at my disposal, I felt that Christine's narrative was meaningful and integrated. Yet, it was only after several sessions of therapy that she could recognize the coherent story she was telling.

THE USEFULNESS OF THIS CONSTRUCTIVIST ACCOUNT OF THERAPY

This account of the constructivist psychology underlying personal construct therapy has been built up through examination of its major assumptions about people and therapy and has concluded with the role of the story in personal construct therapy. It remains to comment on the usefulness of this account. This approach cannot of course be applied by therapists and clients who do not make the constructivist assumptions that I have identified. No theory of psychotherapy can be useful to therapists and clients when the ideas basic to it are not accepted by them. However, a number of theories of psychotherapy do subscribe to many of these assumptions, such as those of some psychodynamic and cognitive-behavioral therapists whom I briefly describe in Chapter 1. However, I now consider in more detail the implications of these ideas for us as therapists as well as for our clients.

READINGS

Psychotherapy Creates Meaning

Bannister, D. (1975). Personal construct theory psychotherapy. In D. Bannister (Ed), *Issues and approaches in the psychological therapies*. London: Wiley.*

Barton, A. (1974). *Three worlds of therapy: Freud, Jung and Rogers*. Palo Alto: National Press Books.

Epting, F. (1981). An appraisal of personal construct psychotherapy. In H. Bonarius, R. Holland, & S. Rosenberg (Eds.), *Personal construct psychology—Recent advances in theory and practice*. London: Macmillan.

Hobson, R.F. (1985). *Forms of feeling*. London: Tavistock.

Viney, L.L. (1981). Experimenting with experience: A psychotherapeutic case study. *Psychotherapy, 18,* 271–278.

Change in the Meaning of Self

Goldfried, M.R. (Ed.). (1982). *Converging themes in psychotherapy*. New York: Springer.

Guidano, U.F. (1991). *A redefinition of cognitive therapy: Using affect in the exploration of self*. New York: Guilford.

Guidano, V.F., & Liotto, G. (1985). A constructivist foundation for cognitive therapy. In M.J. Mahoney & A. Freeman (Eds.), *Cognition and psychotherapy*. New York: Plenum.

Katakis, C.D. (1989). Stages of psychotherapy: Progressive reconceptualizations as a self-organizing process. *Psychotherapy, 26,* 462–468.

Psychotherapy as Constructive Dialogue

Entralgo, P.L. (1970). *The therapy of the word in classical antiquity*. New Haven, CT: Yale University Press.

Hayhow, R., & Levy, C. (1989). *Working with stuttering: A personal construct approach*. Bicester, England: Winslow Press.

---

* Most useful readings.

Joyce-Moniz, L. (1985). Epistemological therapy and constructivism. In M.J. Mahoney & A. Freeman (Eds.), *Cognition and psychotherapy.* New York: Plenum.

Kelly, G.A. (1955). *The psychology of personal constructs.* New York: Norton.*

Kenny, J. (1987). Autopoesis and alternativisim in psychotherapy: Fluctuations and reconstructions. In F. Fransella & L. Thomas (Eds.), *Experimenting with personal construct psychology.* London: Routledge & Kegan Paul.

Lamiell, J.I. (1987). *The psychology of personality: An epistemological enquiry.* New York: Columbia University Press.*

Neimeyer, G.J., & Neimeyer, R.A. (1993). Defining the boundaries of constructivist assessment. In G.J. Neimeyer (Ed.), *Constructivist assessment: A casebook.* New York: Sage.

Schacht, T.E., & Black, D.A. (1985). Epistemological commitments of behavioral and psychoanalytic therapists. *Professional Psychology: Research and Practice, 16,* 316–323.

Winter, D. (1992). *Personal construct psychology in clinical practice.* London: Routledge.

Psychotherapy as Story Telling

Britton, B.K., & Pellegrini, A.D. (1990). *Narrative thought and narrative language.* Hillsdale, NJ: Erlbaum.

Carr, D. (1985). Life and the narrator's art. In H.J. Silverman & D. Ihde (Eds.), *Hermeneutics and deconstruction.* New York: State University of New York Press.

Cohler, B.J. (1982). Personal narrative and life course. In P. Baltes & O.G. Brim (Eds.), *Life span development and behaviour,* (Vol 4). New York: Academic.

Dennett, D.C. (1983). The self as a centre of narrative gravity. In D.L. Johnson & D.M. Cole (Eds.), *Consciousness and self.* New York: Praeger.

Hoshmand, L.T. (1993). The personal narrative in the communal construction of self and life issues. In G. Neimeyer (Ed.), *Constructivist assessment: A casebook.* New York: Sage.*

Kurtzman, H.S. (1987). Deconstruction and psychology: An introduction. *New Ideas in Psychology, 5,* 33–71.

Mair, M. (1989). George Kelly, Don Bannister and a story-telling psychology. *International Journal of Personal Construct Psychology, 2,* 1–14.*

Murphy, G.L., & Medin, D.L. (1985). The role of theories in conceptual coherence. *Psychological Review, 92,* 289–316.

Nash, C. (Ed.). (1990). *Narrative in culture.* New York: Routledge, Chapman & Hall.

Sarbin,T. (Ed.). (1986). *Narrative psychology: The shared nature of human conduct.* New York: Praeger.

Viney, L.L. (1988). Psychotherapy as reconstruction. *International Journal of Personal Construct Psychology. 1,* 30–51.

Viney, L.L. (1993). *Life stories: Personal construct therapy for the elderly.* Chichester: Wiley.

Winter, D.A. (1988). Reconstruing an erection and elaborating ejaculation: Personal construct theory perspective on sex. *International Journal of Personal Construct Psychology, 1,* 81–100.

EXERCISES

1. In successful therapy with a client, describe how his or her construing of self has been changed.
2. The beliefs about how knowledge is created of yourself and a client of yours: Are they similar or different? In what ways?
3. Identify the cohesive and integrating elements of a story of a client of yours. Do they help him or her to function better?
4. Choose a client in crisis, for example, after a rape or a natural disaster. Does he or she lack a story to account for those events?
5. Describe how you and a client have worked together to provide an integrated story for your client. Were the effects of this process therapeutic?

III

CONSTRUING AND RECONSTRUING

4

The Therapist as Construer

In personal construct therapy the constructivist approach to people has many implications for both therapists and clients. In this chapter, I draw attention to therapists as construers, whereas in the next chapter I deal with clients as construers. It is, then, our subjectivity as therapists that is described in this book, our created and shared meanings, and our goals. Our unique and shared meanings are discussed, including those of which we may be, at times, unaware. I am also concerned with our contributions to a psychotherapy that is a dialogue between two construers and in which the stories of those construers are jointly examined. Our stories need to be tested for continuity, as often as those of our clients are. Some of this testing is carried out during therapy but much is conducted before and after it takes place during therapist reflection, supervision, and consultation.

Three major questions about the construing of therapists are answered. First, how do personal construct therapists view therapy? This question is answered in terms of the intentions, experiences, and reflections, as well as in their evaluations of their own developing stories about clients. Second, how do they view their clients? They construe their clients' construing being open to that construing and using their clients' language and metaphors. They also encourage their clients to become joint monitors of the ongoing therapeutic process. Third, how do they view themselves? Therapists need to be aware of themselves as construers. This chapter concludes with consideration of how the construing of therapists changes. Their construing seems to change as a result of both their within-therapy experiences and their personal development outside therapy.

HOW DO THERAPISTS VIEW THERAPY?

Of the intentions, experiences, reflections, and emerging stories of therapists that are examined here, it is the *intentions of therapists* that must be dealt with first. Because these intentions or goals of therapists are central to both the processes and outcomes of therapy, they have been assessed and monitored with some care by researchers (Schmidt, 1984). Such intentions structure experiences of most events, which include therapy (Dalton & Dunnett, 1993). It must even be said that the intentions of therapists can limit the therapy they are able to do (Winter, 1990). When clients have intentions that limit the progress of their therapy, therapists can help them to understand the role this construing is playing so that they can choose to change that construing or not to change it. However, when therapists have such limiting intentions, relatively few of their clients will be able to identify blocks to their progress and work on them (Bannister, 1975). I am responsible for monitoring the effects of my own intentions on therapy. Examples from my therapeutic work with Frank and Christine are again used in this chapter to illustrate my points. It was with Frank that I found I had inappropriately formed the intention of making his indirectly expressed anger unnecessary. No doubt that intention was much related to my own attempts to come to grips with my own expression of anger with a client in therapy. Although I was able to set this old goal of mine to one side, if I had not worked on it in my own therapy I could have interfered early in my relationship with Frank in terms of my understanding of his construing.

Therapists are also responsible for their *experiences* in psychotherapy (Barnes, 1983; Smith, 1979). They listen to and watch their clients, as well as themselves. Yet, they do not remain passive observers. I actively check out my own construing as I encourage my clients to check theirs (Mahrer, 1985; Watzlawick, 1990). As I followed my intentions with Frank, I vigorously pursued his construing of his latest contact with the police. However, as I listened to him attempt to deal with this, I realized just how confused he still was. I then contented myself, for that therapy session at least, with understanding and clarifying his construing of our therapy. To demonstrate to him how I could see us working together, I developed with him an account of his referral, showing how each of us had contributed to the total, coherent referral story.

A *therapist's reflections* are crucial to the processes of personal construct therapy. They try to base their reflections on their experiences of therapy on their careful phenomenological description of what they have experienced in therapy (Fischer, 1985). This means that I explore my construing in several ways (Kelly, 1955, chap. 1 & 4). For example, I identify my own assumptions about people and events and isolate them from those of my client (Winter, 1988). I also try to attend to any culturally shared blind spots I may have. Personal construct therapists will be glad, I am sure, to read in this remark a recommendation for travel, especially to different countries, to test and extend our construct systems. It is only when I have reflected on these experiences that I move on to the constructing of new stories.

Christine's therapy provides an instance. She, with a little encouragement from me, was beginning to talk about her relationship with her father. She claimed that during her childhood and adolescence she had seen relatively little of him and that she "did not feel much about him one way or another." I, as her therapist, reflected on her words. I remembered that I, too, may have said much the same about my father at her age. I did not see much of my father either because he was ill. However, whatever I may have said to myself or anyone else, I would have had some strong feelings of anger and guilt about him. I therefore decided to press Christine further regarding the topic of her father:

Christine: I can remember a few good times with him. He was there when I won my first tennis match. He had been barracking for me, and he was so pleased when I won. His being there just made my day.

Her response showed some of her construing to be like mine and others not to be like mine. It was my reflection that enabled me to make appropriate use of parts of one of my own stories without assuming them all to be true for her.

After therapists have examined their own intentions, observed, and reflected, they are ready to begin to *test the coherence, continuity, and credibility of their own stories* about their clients' worlds (Hobson, 1985; Strohmer & Chiodo, 1984). These stories involve separate elements coming together to form a whole (Schafer, 1980). Stories can even come to link smaller stories in a therapeutic process which is often called interpretation (Frank, 1985). Such story construction is based on experience and reflection. Some of the stories of therapists provide prescriptions for change by clients. The evidence supporting these stories is carefully sought and examined by therapists and unsupported stories are discarded. My own story about psychotherapy as an opportunity to make sense of oneself has been supported in this way.

Christine's description of her father's pleasure at her win at tennis made me wonder whether we may be able to piece together a story for her about her relationship with her father. This story took several therapy sessions to emerge in full:

Christine: He was there when I was born, and he wasn't when any of the other children were. He was a farmer, so once I went to school I saw less of him. But we always knew where we stood with each other. I haven't seen him for a couple of years now.

The story was one of early and continuing closeness between Christine and her father, with a sudden discontinuity brought about by their current separation. I resolved to consider this separation further with Christine.

HOW DO PERSONAL CONSTRUCT THERAPISTS VIEW THEIR CLIENTS?

The primary aim of personal construct therapists is to try to *understand the construing of their clients* (Leitner, 1988). It is not merely their constructs or even their construct systems they pursue. They are concerned with how they make sense of the events they experience (Viney, 1985a). Therapists do not understand the meaning of any statement from their clients until they know the choices it provides, the outcomes it leads to, its context, the experiences of events that led to it, and its importance to clients (Ravenette, 1993). I remember being struck by Frank's sudden outburst of anger against his neighbors in our second session and I wanted to understand his construing of it:

Frank: They are bloody awful. They turn up their radios fucking loud, and I can't get a wink of sleep. They make me so mad. One night I'm going to go down there and kick their door in!

Linda: I can see you are still very angry about it. What did all that noise mean to you?

Frank: Well, my flat is my space and my place . . . and they were coming right inside and taking over. I couldn't hear anything else . . . only them.

One way for therapists to understand the construing of their clients is to try to be *open* to it. Others include using their language and metaphors once they become aware of them. They can even involve their clients as coevaluators of the therapeutic process. The open approach must, however, be understood first. It requires of me as a therapist that I am open to construing events from the vantage point of my clients and into hearing about events through their ears (Epting, 1984). It is by no means easy because my own system of constructs can interfere. I can use a range of methodological techniques to help me listen to my clients (Viney, 1993). Therapeutic openness involves me in accepting clients' construing and, at selected times, even using it instead of my own. It was through my open approach to Frank's anger that we were able to make progress with his recognition and expression of it. I responded to his most recent comments about his neighbors in this way:

Linda: You feel invaded by the noise from your neighbors. It seems to take over, and you want to silence it.

Frank: I hope I won't go and kick their door down. But sometimes I'm afraid I will . . . I just get so angry!

Linda: Is there anything you could do instead which would keep their invasion out? How about doing something that is yours, that they can't take away?

Frank: I don't know . . . I guess there's my radios. I do a lot of tinkering with them in my spare time.

Linda: And you feel that you are doing your own thing in your own place then and keeping your own space.

Frank: Yeah . . .

The openness of personal construct therapists to their clients makes it inappropriate for them to see them as resisting therapy. A client who resists social-skills training is seen as behaving reasonably from the perspective of his or her construct system and the therapist who pushes social-skills training with such a client is seen as failing to be sufficiently open (Winter, 1988).

To aid in their understanding of their clients' construing, personal construct therapists also try to *use some of the language their clients have chosen* (Shapiro, 1979). There is evidence that when therapists and clients start therapy together each uses a different language and that when therapy progresses shared language becomes more common (Winter, 1988). Using some of their clients' language gives therapists an opportunity to experience what it is like for them to talk in a particular way about events. This is partly because the way people use language shapes their experience of events. This shaping has been vividly demonstrated in the types of words people use to talk about physical disease, such as "mounting an attack on a cancer cell" or "marshaling one's forces to ward off a virus" (Viney, 1985b; Warner,

1976–1977). It needs no stretch of the imagination to see how powerful language becomes when dealing with even less tangible psychological problems. However, the power of my clients' language also comes from the way in which people develop individual, often unique languages about their emotions for themselves. I try to develop a working knowledge of each language before I deal with each client. In my most recently reported interaction with Frank about his neighbors, my use of his words "space" and "place" helped me to understand his construing better, as well as aiding him in understanding me.

Therapists can also use *metaphor* as a way of coming to understand the construing of their clients (Mair, 1976). Metaphor involves dealing with one event in terms of another often similar to it in order to explore some of the many possible meanings of that event. Its most common use in therapy is to make more effective comparisons of events possible for both therapists and clients (Siegelman, 1990). Yet, it can be employed to enrich what may otherwise be an inappropriately cognitive comparison with its appropriate emotions (Combs & Freedman, 1990). It can also be used to ignore irrelevancies in comparisons that may be distracting (Lakoff & Johnson, 1980).

The most effective metaphors I manage to choose as a therapist are those of sufficient complexity to do justice to the complexity of the events they represent (Gordon, 1978). Metaphors are also created meanings and as such they help me to show my clients their abilities as construers. In my interaction with Frank about his anger at his neighbors, I used the metaphor of "invasion" to represent something of his experience of their noise. It was my metaphor and not his but I chose it partly because of Frank's interest in military things. The metaphor also seemed suited to his emotional reaction to it; his wanting to "kick their door in." By using this invasion metaphor, I was able to achieve many of the therapeutic functions of metaphor, such as providing Frank with a comparison with other threats which was appropriately complex and emotion laden. It also served me as a device for testing my understanding of Frank's construing and, as it proved, showing my understanding to him.

Therapists understand their clients' construing best when they see them as *joint monitors with them* of the therapeutic process. This shared role is very similar to that of the client as coevaluator during psychological assessment (Fischer, 1970). When clients are seen as coevaluators, they work together with the therapist to develop a joint account of their referral, which also involves sharing expectations of therapy (Fischer, 1985). To make this sharing possible, I try to use everyday language as much as is feasible and not my sometimes more customary psychological jargon. As I have shown, clients have an important role in monitoring the therapeutic process. It was very difficult for Frank to take on this monitoring role. Many of my constructs about psychotherapy were alien to him, like my assumption that talking about problems helps, although they would be very familiar to other therapists. Like Christine, he especially found any suggestion that he take some responsibility for what happened in his therapy difficult to handle. Our setting of the five-session limit on the number of therapy sessions that we would have helped him to see that he would need to work to identify his own unresolved issues or we may find ourselves wasting our opportunities. It also gave him the chance to use his language rather than mine to describe our contract.

HOW DO THERAPISTS VIEW THEMSELVES?

It follows from these constructivist assumptions about therapy that therapists must be concerned with how they *monitor their own therapy-related construing and actions* (Kelly, 1955, chap. 1 & 4). Expectations about therapy are usually seen as influencing clients rather than therapists; yet, their impact on therapists is equally important (Kenny, 1988, pp. 140–147). Had Christine been older, therapists working with her could have found their therapeutic effects interfered with by their own expectations of the client. When working with the elderly the use of disempowering expectations has to be very often monitored (Viney, 1993). These expectations come from the lives of us therapists, but also from our training and professional experience. Generally, they help to maintain therapist self-esteem and to develop relationships with clients. My successful piecing together of Christine's story about her father and my recognition of its sudden discontinuity helped both to maintain my view of myself as an effective therapist and to make me feel closer to Christine whom I was coming to understand better. It had led me off into my stories about my own father but I was not sidetracked by them. How do therapists achieve this self-monitoring?

The meanings that emerge from the therapeutic interaction need to be valid and useful for both therapists and clients. A subsuming construct system has been required of these therapists (Kelly, 1955, chap. 1 & 4). A subsuming system is one that should work effectively with the construing of a wide range of clients. Therapists' construct systems help them to make sense of those of their clients and not simply provide an alternative view to theirs. One way to improve the chances of this occurring is for therapists to test their construing of clients in supervisory discussions with other therapists who may be either teachers or peers (Blumenfied, 1982; Hess, 1980). When beginning therapy, I always ask my clients for permission to consult at least one other appropriate person about our therapy. I needed to be able, then, to make sense of both Christine's and Frank's systems of constructs in order to be able to work therapeutically with each of them. Yet, clients' construing can differ from one another's much more than the construing of those two did and even more from that of their therapist. It may well be that the people who come for psychotherapy are those whose construing is least understood by the people around them so that they present a special challenge to therapists.

HOW DOES THE CONSTRUING OF THERAPISTS CHANGE?

Before therapists become too confident about their ability to monitor their own construing, it is important for them to recognize that the *construing of therapists is continually changing* (Kelly, 1955, chap. 1 & 4). It changes in the course of therapy with each client, as my work with Christine and Frank reported in this chapter has shown. Yet, it also changes with my accumulated experiences of working with different clients. When I enter therapy with them, my construing of myself and other people and events may change. Over the years of intimately sharing the experiences of clients, my construct system enables me to make sense of a wide range of other types of construing, but it also continues to change. For example, I have come to see my clients as having at least as much to offer in therapy as I do. Ideally, this process of change never stops for even the most mature of therapists. However, being available to change through taking an open approach to clients, for example, is very demanding. There are many times when I am not as open to changes in my construing as I would like. Sometimes this is because I am not as open to the construing of some clients as I would like. It is then that consultation with other therapists who can be open to them is useful to me.

Some changes in therapist construing are due to the *personal development of the therapist*. The constructivist approach to psychological development maintains that consecutive experiences are interpreted and reinterpreted by people throughout their life span, with the result that they accumulate a wider range of constructs as they have more experiences (Viney, 1992). This wider range of constructs does not necessarily come with advancing age but with experience with certain age-related tasks. I have learned much about my own strengths (and something of my own weaknesses) in maintaining a close relationship in the last 20 years. There is evidence that younger people use constructs that deal with earlier age-related tasks, such as experiencing autonomy and developing a sense of identity, whereas older people use both these constructs and those relating to later tasks, such as generativity and integrity (Viney, 1987). In these tasks, they come to nurture and support others and develop a sense of the worth of their lives and an acceptance of themselves. Therapists will, in the main, tend to use construing that is appropriate to the psychological tasks of their age group. This tendency can lead to problems when therapists are trying to understand the construing of clients in age groups different from theirs. I manage to recall some of my earlier constructs effectively when I am working with younger clients but I have more difficulty in anticipating constructs I have used very little when I work with elderly clients (Viney, Benjamin, & Preston, 1992). Generally, however, these personal developmental changes in my construing should permit me to be a better therapist because as I make them I am extending and elaborating my own construct system. This process involves some distress from the invalidation of some of my constructs, but disconfirmation and discomfort is ultimately of benefit to both myself and to my clients.

THERAPISTS AS CONSTRUERS

The need to monitor the construing of therapists that is recognized by this personal construct therapy suggests that two acts of therapists are particularly important. The first of these is personal reflection on the implications of their stories about therapy, their clients, and themselves. The second is their sharing of these stories with therapy supervisors or colleagues who are experienced therapists to ensure that their necessary subjectivity does not blind them to those implications. Therapists, then, are construers, but are clients? In the next chapter I answer this question.

READING NOTES

How Do Therapists View Therapy?

Bannister, D. (1975). Personal construct theory psychotherapy. In D. Bannister (Ed.), *Issues and approaches in the psychological therapies*. London: Wiley.

Barnes, B. (1983). Doubts and certainties in practising psychotherapy. In D. Pilgrim (Ed.), *Psychology and psychotherapy*. London: Routledge & Kegan Paul.

Dalton, S., & Dunnett, G. (1993). *Living personal construct psychology.* Chichester: Wiley.
Fischer, C.T. (1985). *Individualizing psychological assessment.* Monterey, CA: Brooks/Cole.
Frank, J. (1985). Therapeutic components shared by all psychotherapies. In M.J. Mahoney & A. Freeman (Eds.), *Cognition and psychotherapy.* New York: Plenum.
Hobson, R.F. (1985). *Forms of feeling.* London: Tavistock.
Kelly, G.A. (1955). *The psychology of personal constructs.* New York: Norton.*
Mahrer, A.H. (1985). *Psychotherapeutic change.* New York: Norton.
Schafer, R. (1980). Narration in the psychoanalytic dialogue. *Critical Enquiry, 7,* 29–53.
Schmidt, J. (1984). Counsellor intentionality: An emerging view of process and performance. *Journal of Counselling Psychology, 31,* 383–386.
Smith, D.L. (1979). Phenomenological psychotherapy: A why and how. In A. Giorgi, R. Knowles, & D.L. Smith (Eds.), *Duquesne studies in phenomenological psychology* (Vol. 3). Pittsburgh: Duquesne University Press.
Strohmer, D.C., & Chiodo, A.L. (1984). Counsellor hypothesis testing strategies: The role of initial impressions and self schema. *Journal of Counselling Psychology, 31,* 510–519.
Watzlawick, P. (1990). *Munchausen's pigtail.* London: Norton.
Winter, D. (1988). Towards a constructive clinical psychology. In G. Dunnett (Ed.), *Working with people.* London: Routledge.
Winter, D.A. (1990). Therapeutic alternatives for psychological disorders: Personal construct psychology investigations in a health service setting. In G.J. & R.A. Neimeyer (Eds.), *Advances in personal construct psychology* (Vol. 1). Greenwich, CT: JAI.

How do Therapists View Their Clients?

Combs, G., & Freedman, J. (1990). *Symbol, story and ceremony: Using metaphor in individual and family therapy.* London: Norton.
Epting, F.R. (1984). *Personal construct counselling and psychotherapy.* Chichester: Wiley.
Fischer, C.T. (1970). The testee as co-evaluator. *Journal of Counselling Psychology, 17,* 70–76.
Gordon, D. (1978). *Therapeutic metaphors.* Cupertino, CA: Meta.
Lakoff, G., & Johnson, M. (1980). *Metaphors we live by.* Chicago: University of Chicago Press.
Leitner, L.M. (1988). Terror, risk and reverence: Experiential personal construct psychotherapy. *International Journal of Personal Construct Psychology, 1,* 251–262.
Mair, M. (1976). Metaphors for living. *Nebraska Symposium on Motivation, 24,* 243—290.*

---

* Most useful readings.

Ravenette, A.T. (1993, July). *Asking questions within a personal construct framework.* Paper presented at the meeting of the 10th International Personal Construct Congress, Townsville, Australia.
Shapiro, T. (1979). *Clinical psycholinguistics.* London: Plenum.
Siegelman, E.Y. (1990). *Metaphor and meaning in psychotherapy.* New York: Guilford.
Viney, L.L. (1985a). Humour as a therapeutic tool. In A. Landfield & F. Epting (Eds.), *Anticipating personal construct theory.* Lincoln: University of Nebraska Press.
Viney, L.L. (1985b). Physical illness: A guidebook for the kingdom of the sick. In E. Button (Ed.), *Personal construct theory and mental health.* Beckenham: Croom Helm.
Viney, L.L. (1993). Listening to what my clients say: Content analysis categories and scales. In G.J. Neimeyer (Ed.), *Casebook of constructivist assessment.* New York: Sage.
Warner, R. (1976–1977). The relationship between language and disease concepts. *International Journal of Psychiatry in Medicine, 7,* 57–78.
Winter, D. (1988). PCP: A radical alternative to social skills training. In P. Maitland (Ed.), *Personal construct theory, deviancy and social work.* London: Inner London Probation Service and the Centre for Personal Construct Psychology.

How do Therapists View Themselves?

Blumenfied, M.D. (Ed.). (1982). *Applied supervision in psychotherapy.* New York: Grune & Stratton.
Hess, A.K. (Ed.). (1980). *Psychotherapy supervision: Theory, research and practice.* Chichester: Wiley.
Kenny, J. (1988). Changing conversations: A constructivist model of training for psychotherapists. In G. Dunnett (Ed.), *Working with people: Clinical uses of personal construct psychology.* London: Routledge.*
Viney, L.L. (1993). *Life stories: Personal construct therapy for the elderly.* Chichester: Wiley.

How Does the Construing of Therapists Change?

Viney, L.L. (1987). A sociophenomenological approach to life span development complementing Erikson's psychodynamic approach. *Human Development, 30,* 125–136.
Viney, L.L. (1992). Can we see ourselves changing?: Toward a constructivist model of adult lifespan development. *Human Development, 36,* 65–75.*
Viney, L.L., Benjamin, Y.N., & Preston, C. (1992). Personal construct therapy for the elderly. *International Journal of Cognitive Therapy, 4,* 27–40.

EXERCISES

1. Identify some of your most important interventions with a client. Do they fit with or compete with the therapeutic goals that you two have expressed?
2. Describe a construct of a client. What choices do its twin poles provide? To what outcomes does it lead? When does he or she use it? What earlier events led to its creation? Is it important to your client?
3. Choose a metaphor that you have used with a client that was helpful. In what ways did it help?
4. Can you use parts of your construct system to make sense of that of your client? When this is difficult what can you do to aid this process?
5. Listen to your own speech to see if you are using constructs that are appropriate to your age group and life tasks. Show how this can make your understanding of a client older than you difficult.

5

The Client as Construer

If it is important for those of us who take a constructivist view of therapy to consider therapists as construers of meaning, it is equally important for us to consider our clients as construers. To undergo the discipline of seeing myself as a therapist in the role of the active creator of meanings has served to promote my own self-awareness. However, to discipline myself sufficiently to view my clients in that role is to attempt to bridge the gap between their personal meanings and my own. Their construing is often more difficult to understand than that of therapists in at least two ways. The content of their construing of self can be demeaning and belittling to them in ways that interfere with their attempts at therapy. Also, the structure of their construct systems can be chaotic with their construing so confused that they cannot even form a relationship with their therapist. I need, then, to think carefully about my clients as construers.

In this chapter, I raise three questions about the construing of clients. These questions have the same foci as those that I have considered for therapists. First, how do my clients view therapy? Their construing is, like that of therapists, influenced by the myths about therapy available to them. These myths can be helpful or misleading. Therapy also involves clients in being confronted with personal meanings they may want to avoid. Clients need help to construe therapy. Second, how do my clients view me as a therapist? Initially, this viewing is with anxiety and therapists are seen as in control of the therapy. However, as my clients come to understand my understanding of their understanding, I can help them reformulate their own meanings. Third, how do my clients view themselves? I deal with their construing of themselves and of losses of parts of their worlds. I also examine the continuity and content of their stories. Something of how I assess my clients' construing of themselves is demonstrated and the continual changes in the construing of clients, like those of therapists, are considered.

HOW DO CLIENTS VIEW THERAPY?

Myths About Therapy

Clients view therapy in a multitude of ways, far too many to consider here. However, it is worth looking at some of their main ways. They may have been exposed to myths about therapy, which could either aid or frustrate the therapeutic process (Dunnett, 1988, pp. 1–16). They also see therapy as confronting them with some of the meanings of therapeutic myths of which they have been unaware. I therefore need to help my clients to construe their therapy in ways that will contribute to our therapeutic process.

Many *helpful effects of clients' myths* or stories about therapy that have not been tested have been identified (Barton, 1974). Myths may, for example, strengthen the therapeutic relationship by allowing clients to anticipate the actions of their therapists in positive ways. They can encourage expectations of help and therefore, of hopefulness. They enable clients to try out the therapeutic learning process before therapy starts and offer opportunities for clients to rehearse their approaches. Christine had heard a few positively orienting myths about psychotherapy from a high-school teacher who had suggested that she may find it useful. The teacher had supported Christine through a time of crisis; of which more will be revealed later. The teacher's description of therapy was essentially mythical because she had never experienced it herself. However, her myths enabled Christine to begin to relate well to me as her therapist, even before we met, and to hope for good things from our relationship. It was these positive expectations that enabled Christine to appear for her first interview, even though she was at the same time condemning herself as weak and pitiable because she felt that she needed therapy.

Myths about therapy can also hinder the therapeutic process (Kelly, 1955, chap. 3 & 11). For me, this can occur if a client has accepted misleading myths about therapy that require acceptance of assumptions that are not compatible with my constructivist approach. An example of such an assumption would be a client seeing his or her meanings as given to him or her rather than created by him- or herself. Myths about therapy also can be misleading when they assign roles to therapists and clients that are not compatible with personal construct therapy, such as doctors and patients or priests and penitents (Bannister, 1983). Frank, once he had moved from his view of our roles as doctor and patient, took up another of his myths to see me as teacher and student. For me, as a university-based teacher with a history of many rewarding experiences of relationships with students, this was helpful. For Frank, however, as a man with a history of poor studentship with most of his school teachers, it was not. He began to construe my role to be authoritarian and even punitive until we were able to achieve a relationship that could be more therapeutic for him.

Therapy as Confrontation and Confusion

Therapy may be confronting to clients. Clients may well have remained unaware of certain meanings affecting their lives until they come to therapy. Thus, therapy may become an arena in which they are confronted with the need to change those meanings, and it can then come to constitute a threat to them (Benbenishty & Schul, 1987). There was such an event in Christine's life with which her therapy did confront her. The discontinuity of the story of her relationship with her father pointed to it. It was when she was 15 years old that she first had sexual intercourse with her boyfriend, who later became her husband. Her parents, as soon as they knew this, assumed that she was pregnant. She ran away from home when they condemned her and had interacted very little with them since that time. This event caused her relationship with her father to be disrupted and also the crisis that brought her close to one of her teachers. Her confrontation with that event in therapy was painful but opened up ways for her to change.

Clients may need help to construe therapy. Personal construct therapy involves a unique therapeutic process and a unique therapeutic relationship. It is not possible for clients to come to a useful construing of it before they are involved in it. It is therefore appropriate for therapists to spend some time in therapy helping them to construe it. This must be done, of course, within the range of the construct systems of their clients (Bannister & Fransella, 1986). I need to make sense of what I am doing in therapy in their terms. This involves a sharing of those constructs about therapy that I have identified as constructivist. My clients need to come to understand that during therapy we will be creating meanings and that these meanings have to do with their views of themselves (Viney, 1989). These meanings will be created through our constructive dialogue. In communicating these constructs, professional jargon is not used. Indeed, often it is my actions rather than my words that convey these messages. Given Frank's frustrating choice of roles for us as client and therapist, and his preference for action over words, I found that I could best convey the possibilities of a constructive dialogue with him by getting into such dialogue with him.

HOW DO MY CLIENTS VIEW THEIR THERAPISTS?

Clients view their therapists, initially at least, with *anxiety*. They see their therapists as in control, so that clients often do try to understand some of the construing of their therapists. When that occurs, it is possible for therapists to become reconstruers of meanings in the eyes of their clients.

When my clients first meet me, they often know little about me. The *confusion* of their construing of me is likely to be joined by anxiety generated by the unpredictability of my actions for them (Leitner, 1990). Such anxiety can also arise from conflicts within their own construct system (Leitner, 1985). Such anxiety is likely, also, to be considerable if these clients have tended to limit their dependency to a very small range of people (Chiaro et al., 1994). Those clients with undispersed dependencies will have difficulty in extending them to a therapist. Christine, for example, asked nothing about me during our early sessions. This was probably because she chose to meet a standard of politeness that I would have shared with her had we met under other circumstances. Then she became overtly interested in my life away from therapy:

Christine: I probably shouldn't ask this, but . . . are you married?

Linda: Yes.

Christine: I suppose you get on pretty well with your husband?

Linda: Yes, but I know what it's like to have him busy with his own things when I feel I need him. I think every couple has that problem from time to time.

My anticipation that she wanted validation and even sharing of her feelings of rejection seemed to be a useful one because she returned to explore her feelings in that area more fully and very rarely again moved from her experience to mine. The one exception to this in later sessions was, of course, in my feelings about her.

Control is currently a central issue in psychotherapy process research and it would seem that clients often see their therapists as more in control of what happens in therapy than they are (Friedlander & Schwartz, 1985). This research literature provides evidence that as therapy progresses, clients work to gain more control; however, there is no evidence to suggest that therapy with therapists in control rather than clients is more successful (Friedlander & Schwartz, 1985). Although clients may need to see therapists as in control when they begin therapy, therapists are usually eager to change this view (Fischer & Fischer, 1983). My intentions usually are that my clients will emerge from their therapy with an enhanced sense of personal control. Personal construct therapy works to empower clients in their social contexts. For Frank, control in therapy was a very important issue. Although he would often appear to give control to me, as his doctor or teacher, any action of mine that he perceived as loosening his control of the content of our sessions was seen as a threat and was responded to with anger and anxiety.

Clients try to construe the construing of therapists. Although clients may sometimes see therapists as threatening, they also try to understand and anticipate how they are thinking and feeling about them (Kelly, 1955, chap. 3 & 11). It is, of course, the responsibility of therapists to make this possible. Yet, from a constructivist viewpoint, there is much that stands in the way of such an understanding. As a therapist, for example, I have superordinate constructs influencing much of my own construing that may be quite different from those of my clients. I may also use different words to express our construing from those of my clients. Eventually, I can come to reconstrue my client's stories with them but not until some assumptions and words that are common to both of us have been established. Frank could come to understand something of my construing of his therapy as a reconstructive dialogue from my actual engagement in dialogue with him. Yet, his understanding was much extended by my finding a language with which I could communicate with him better. This proved, in his case, to be a language based on concrete rather than abstract ideas.

Therapists are changers of meanings. Clients also come to view therapists as validators and changers of meanings (G.J. Neimeyer, 1987). They come to therapy with one set of personal meanings and leave it with choices between a wider range of meanings (Button, 1994). The meanings that are changed and elaborated in therapy often have to do with their construing of self. Although clients are in part themselves responsible for these changes, they often tend to attribute them to their therapists. Christine saw me as a reconstruer of meanings when we dealt with her break with her family. She was much hurt by their unjust accusation of her because she was not pregnant and had taken appropriate precautions. Yet, she had not dealt directly with her feelings of rejection by them. After she did so in therapy she was able to move onto some new meanings for herself and them:

Christine: I can understand, now, why they jumped to conclusions. I was a typical teenager. No one knew what was going on inside me. And they had the rest of the family to worry about. I just feel sad that we have been apart for so long. . . . Maybe I'll go and see them.

HOW DO CLIENTS VIEW THEMSELVES?

Much has been learned about the content of clients' construing of themselves (Beail, 1985; Button, 1985), and only a small portion of it can be reported here. I deal with their construing of themselves and their worlds, especially in relation to how they make sense of the loss of loved ones. The continuity and discontinuity of their stories is examined, as well as how their construing is assessed by personal construct therapists.

Clients' Construing of Themselves and Their Worlds

The *construing of clients* with many different types of presenting psychological problems has been examined. These problems include depression, eating disorders, other neuroses, psychoses, alcoholism, and other drug-addictive disorders (R.A. Neimeyer, 1985). The construing of people in general hospitals and jails has been examined, as has that of those who are developmentally disabled. Some of the most useful work of this kind has contrasted the construing of these people with that of people whose psychological functioning is good. Generally speaking, the construing of the people who become psychotherapy clients is more pessimistic in content and more poorly organized. It is beyond the scope of this book to consider their construing in detail but depressive construing will serve to illustrate these general trends.

The construing of depressed clients has been characterized as constricted (Rowe, 1989). That constriction is apparent in both the content of their constructs and in their use. Depressives' construing of themselves is negatively based and they see themselves as alienated from others. They have difficulty in anticipating a future for themselves and when they manage to do so their construing of their future is also negatively toned (Sheehan, 1985). Christine showed all these types of depressive construing during her initial therapy sessions. She saw herself as incompetent and unlovable and perceived herself to be alienated from her parents and, to a lesser extent, her husband. She could not at first speculate on her own future but when she did her predictions were sad and self-defeating. She was, however, eventually able, by some courageous acts, to loosen some of the constriction in her construing.

How clients construe their worlds can best be shown by considering what happens when they lose an important part of it. Most clients have experienced some losses. Yet, it is not only the loss of loved ones in the world that leads to mourning; mourning of any part of their world can cause them to lose their usual sources of confirmation for their construing. Mourning has been extensively examined by constructivists (Epting & Neimeyer, 1983; R. A. Neimeyer & Epting, 1992). They have concluded that mourning does not necessarily occur in objectively viewed consecutive stages, as has been claimed by those with nonconstructivist views, but in the subjective concurrently occurring processes of dislocation and adaptation of construing (Woodfield & Viney, 1985). Dislocated construing in clients results in their failing to anticipate new events effectively. Adaptive construing can occur, however, if in therapy clients can come to change either the events or the constructs involved in their construing to achieve better functioning (Viney, 1990).

Frank showed all these coexisting processes of dislocation and adaptation in his reaction to his recent loss of his job. His job record had not been good but he had been able to get casual laboring jobs when he wanted them. Yet, it had been made clear to him that he was no longer well enough for such jobs and so he was forced to give up his view of himself as a paid worker. His construing was, as a result, dislocated so that he could not effectively predict his own future: "I don't know what's to become of me." However, at the same time Frank's attempts at some form of adaptation to his new world were apparent. His angry denial of his loss of physical fitness demonstrated his attempts to change the events of his world: "They don't know what they're talking about, the silly buggers! I'm still as fit as ever." His suspicious anxiety about his new situation showed that he was testing some changes to his constructs: "I don't know what's going on either. Maybe they've got it in for me."

Clients' Stories, Their Continuity, and Content

Clients present themselves to their therapists through the stories they tell (Hoshmand, 1993). Their stories represent themselves and their worlds. Such stories serve as the means by which they organize their thoughts, feelings, wishes, intentions, and actions (Viney, 1993). When therapists listen to their clients' stories, they check that this organizing function is effective. Yet, they also listen for the content of their stories because this content will guide their construing. Good continuity in the stories of clients can represent not only good organization of themselves and their worlds, but also an effective integration of past, present, and future (Viney & Bousfield, 1992). There are times, however, when this integration needs to be loose. In personal construct therapy, as in stories, time is transcended. Clients and therapists neither focus on the past, nor the here and now, nor on anticipations of the future alone, but on integrations of past, present and future as it is represented in the construing of clients (Combs & Freedman, 1990).

The content of clients' stories may take the major forms available in the literature of romance, tragedy, or irony, depending on the pessimism of their ending. They may also develop self-defeating stories. Clients with certain kinds of problems tend to produce certain kinds of stories; for example, clients with paranoid concerns develop stories that go beyond mere tragedy to the end of both self and world. Frank proved to be living with a story with something of this cataclysmic character. It emerged in many discontinuous fragments and served only poorly to organize his constructs. He believed that his world would eventually end in a nuclear holocaust. He saw these hostile forces as building up from the time of World War I and occasionally had glimpses of how he personally may come to an end in a great fire.

Other Assessments of Clients' Construing

The *main techniques used to assess the construing of clients* by personal construct therapists are now considered. Their assessments have been of the organization and content of their clients' stories (G.J. Neimeyer, 1993), although these techniques have been referred to as assessments of disorders of construction and transition (Kelly, 1955, chap. 3 & 11). Disorders of construction refer to problems in how clients make sense of their worlds. Disorders of transition refer to problems of disconfirmation of construing and so need to change. The Repertory Grid Technique has been most often used for this purpose but it is not always used in a manner compatible with constructivist assumptions (Bell, 1988). Its results have tended to be both oversimplified and static rather than complex and dynamic. There is, however, a wide range of other techniques for finding out about the content our clients' worlds, such as eliciting accounts of significant life events, laddering, and pyramiding (Hayhow & Levy, 1989). Laddering involves repeatedly asking the question "Why?" about the use of a positive construct pole so as to discover the most influential meanings people have in their construct systems. Pyramiding involves asking the question "How?" about the use of a particular construct pole in order to find the context in which it is asked. The most fruitful of these techniques may well be self-characterization, in which clients write a description of themselves from an external but sympathetic viewpoint (Fransella, 1981). There are also techniques for assessing the organization of their construing: for example, its flexibility, control, and sources of validation (R.A. Neimeyer, 1993). I provide more information about these assessment devices in Chapter 8. Such assessment continues throughout therapy and is not used only before therapy starts. It is also likely to become during therapy a shared responsibility rather than being solely that of the therapist.

All of these constructivist techniques for assessing the construing of clients are useful not only for assessment, but also because they often begin the therapeutic processes (Leitner, 1985). Clients who reflect jointly with me on how they see their worlds are on the way to recognizing that they create those images themselves. This was apparent in therapy with Christine. I was using one of my customary methods for identifying a clients' constructs. In other words, I was making a thematic analysis of the contents of what she said to me. As I listened to her talk about feeling "socially isolated," I wondered what the opposite pole of this construct was for her. Because she was focusing on the negative side of things, no trace of the other construct pole appeared in her speech. As her depression lifted a little, she was able to indulge herself in a fantasy about not being socially isolated, whom she would be with, and what she would do. It proved that the opposite of "socially isolated" for her was "socially involved and useful." She was then able to test this regained bipolar construing of herself by going back to coach a young team of basketball players. This was an activity she had given up as her depression increased but now was able to enjoy.

HOW DO THE CONSTRUCTS OF CLIENTS CHANGE?

As for therapists, the construing of clients is changing continually. It changes during each psychotherapy session, as I have already indicated. It also changes within the course of therapy and as a result of personal development. These latter, more major types of changes are now discussed.

Some changes occur as a result of the *experience of therapy.* A range of changes is experienced by clients as they move successfully through their therapy (Fransella, 1985). These include changes in their central assumptions about themselves and their worlds and how to change them, as well as in the content of their constructs and the way in which they are organized (R.A. Neimeyer & Harter, 1988). They also include changes in the way they use language and in their emotional states. It follows that during each therapy session, therapists must listen very attentively to their clients in order to keep up with these changes. Therapists should not assume that their initial assessments of their psychological functioning are still appropriate.

Some changes occur as a result of the *personal development of clients*. Clients, like therapists, are continually construing events that are important to them and the events with which they deal vary throughout the entire life span. This means that they may be, as therapists work with them, in the process of adding a new set of constructs appropriate to the developmental tasks of their age group to their construct systems (Viney, 1987). If so, therapists can then work with them to achieve this addition. Its other implication, however, provides more food for thought. Clients in different age groups use some very different constructs. Indeed, they should do so if their psychological growth has been similar to that of others of their age group. Can therapists, at a particular point in their life spans, deal effectively with such construing? Child therapists have learned to work within the constraints on construing that their clients have, but then they have already construed in those limited ways themselves. I have tried to find special ways of understanding those clients, some of which I have described in Chapter 6.

CLIENTS AS CONSTRUERS

In this chapter, the need for personal construct therapists to understand the construing of their clients has been recognized. My original set of questions about construing, which were asked about therapists in Chapter 4, has here been asked about clients. The issues relevant to those questions have been examined. How do clients view their therapy? Even before they come to therapy they have learned myths about it, some facilitating good psychotherapy, others not. Clients can see therapy as confronting them with meanings that they have been avoiding. They clearly need help from us therapists in their construing of therapy. How do clients view their therapists? Initially, because of a lack of information they view them with anxiety, but then as the person whose construing must be made sense of, therapists become reconstruers of their meanings. How do clients view themselves? I have considered the content of their construing of self and world together with its organization. The content and continuity of their stories has been examined. The means by which this construing of clients is assessed have also been discussed.

The other major theme of this chapter has been the changeability and variability of the construing of clients. These characteristics come as no surprise to personal construct therapists, for whom all human experience is continually changing. This capacity to change is especially important to the ideas in my next chapter, in which I examine the implications of the constructivist assumption that the essential ingredient of psychotherapy is reconstruction.

READINGS

How Do Clients View Therapy?

Bannister, D. (1983). The internal politics of psychotherapy. In D. Pilgrim (Ed.), *Psychology and psychotherapy.* London: Routledge & Kegan Paul.

Bannister, D., & Fransella, F. (1986). *Inquiring man.* Beckenham: Croom Helm.

Barton, A. (1974). *Three worlds of therapy: Freud, Jung and Rogers.* Palo Alto, CA: National Press Books.

Benbenishty, R., & Schul, Y. (1987). Client–therapist congruence of expectations over the course of therapy. *British Journal of Clinical Psychology, 26,* 17–24.

Dunnett, G. (1988). Myths, methods and techniques. In G. Dunnett (Ed.), *Working with people.* London: Routledge.*

Kelly, G.A. (1955). *The psychology of personal constructs.* New York: Norton.

Viney, L.L. (1989). *Images of illness.* Malabar, FL: Krieger.

How Do Clients View Their Therapists?

Button, E. (1994). *Personal construct therapy for eating disorders.* Chichester: Wiley.

Chiaro, G., Nuzzo, L., Alfano, V., Brogna, P., D'Andrea, T., Di Battista, G., Plata, P., & Stefan, G. (1994). Personal paths of dependency. *International Journal of Personal Construct Psychology, 7,* 112–122.

Fischer, C.T., & Fischer, W.F. (1983). Phenomenological–existential psychotherapy. In M. Hersen, A.E. Kazdin, & A.S. Bellack (Eds.), *The clinical psychology handbook.* New York: Pergamon.

Friedlander, M.L., & Schwartz, G.S. (1985). Toward a theory of strategic self-presentation in counselling and psychotherapy. *Journal of Counselling Psychology, 32,* 483–501.

---

* Most useful readings.

Leitner, L.M. (1985). The terrors of cognition: On the experiential validity of personal construct theory. In D. Bannister (Ed.), *Issues and approaches in personal construct theory.* London: Academic.*

Leitner, L.M. (1990). Terror, risk and reverence: Experiential personal construct psychotherapy. *International Journal of Personal Construct Psychology, 3,* 28–39.

Neimeyer, G.J. (1987). Personal construct assessment, strategy and technique. In R.A. Neimeyer & G.J. Neimeyer (Eds.), *Personal construct therapy casebook.* New York: Springer.

How Do Clients View Themselves?

Beail, N. (1985). *Repertory grid technique in personal constructs: Applications in clinical and educational settings.* London: Croom Helm.

Bell, R.C. (1988). Theory appropriate analyses of Repertory Grid data. *International Journal of Personal Construct Psychology, 1,* 126–138.

Button, E. (Ed.). (1985). *Personal construct theory and mental health.* London: Croom Helm.

Combs, G., & Freedman, J. (1990). *Symbol, story and ceremony: Using metaphor in individual and family therapy.* London: Norton.

Epting, F., & Neimeyer, R.A. (Eds.). (1983). *Personal meanings of death.* Washington, D.C.: Hemisphere.

Fransella, F. (1981). Nature babbling to herself: The self-characterisation as a therapeutic tool. In H. Bonarius, R. Holland & S. Rosenberg (Eds.), *Personal construct psychology: Recent advances in theory and practice.* New York: St. Martin's Press.

Hayhow, R., & Levy, C. (1989). *Working with stuttering: A personal construct approach.* Bicester, England: Winslow Press.

Hoshmand, L.T. (1993). The personal narrative in the construction of self and life issues. In G.J. Neimeyer (Ed.), *Constructivist assessment: A case book.* New York: Sage.

Leitner, L.M. (1985). Interview methodologies for construct elicitation: Searching for the core. In F. Epting & A.W. Landfield (Eds.), *Anticipating personal construct psychology.* Lincoln: University of Nebraska Press.

Neimeyer, G.J. (Ed.). (1993). *Constructivist assessment: A casebook.* New York: Sage.

Neimeyer, R.A. (1985). Personal constructs in clinical practice. In P.C. Kendall (Ed.), *Advances in cognitive-behavioural research and therapy.* New York: Academic.*

Neimeyer, R.A. (1993). Constructivist approaches to the measurement of meaning. In G.J. Neimeyer (Ed.), *Constructivist assessment: A casebook.* New York: Sage.*

Neimeyer, R.A., & Epting, F.R. (1992). Measuring personal meanings of death: Twenty years of research using the Threat Index. In R.A. & G.J. Neimeyer (Eds.), *Advances in personal construct psychology.* Greenwich, CT: JAI.

Rowe, D. (1989). *Depression: The way out of your prison.* London: Routledge.

Sheehan, M.J. (1985). Personal construct theory and depression. *British Journal of Medical Psychology, 33,* 2–14.
Viney, L.L. (1990). The construing widow: Dislocation and adaptation in bereavement. *Psychotherapy Patient, 3,* 207–222.
Viney, L.L. (1993). *Life stories: Personal construct therapy for the elderly.* Chichester: Wiley.
Viney, L.L., & Bousfield, L. (1992). AIDS and the client "in the fast lane": Narrative construction and reconstruction. *The Psychotherapy Patient, 8,* 141–156.
Woodfield, R.L., & Viney, L.L. (1985). A personal construct approach to bereavement. *Omega, 16,* 1–13.

How Do The Constructs Of Clients Change?

Fransella, F. (1985). Individual psychotherapy. In E. Button (Ed.), *Personal construct theory and mental health.* Beckenham: Croom Helm.*
Neimeyer, R.A., & Harter, S. (1988). Facilitating individual change in personal construct therapy. In G. Dunnett (Ed.), *Personal construct psychology in clinical settings.* London: Routledge & Kegan Paul.
Viney, L.L. (1987). A sociophenomenological approach to life span development complementing Erikson's psychodynamic approach. *Human Development, 30,* 125–136.

EXERCISES

1. Describe how you go about making the processes of therapy meaningful for a client.
2. Consider how at least two of your clients see you as a therapist. Are there similarities in their views? Are there differences? Which of your clients' constructs have led to these differences?
3. Select a client of yours who is experiencing depression. How does he or she use his or her constructs and what is their content? Are these constructs used in a constricted way? Is their content negative and alienated with few anticipations of the future?
4. Select a client of yours who is grieving. Can you detect the dislocation in his or her construct system?
5. With this client or another, consider whether he or she is using constructs that are appropriate to his or her age group and life tasks. If the answer is no, how is this problematic for the daily life of your client?

6

Reconstruction in Personal Construct Therapy

I have provided accounts of the therapists and clients involved in personal construct therapy as construers. It is now time to turn to the heart of this approach, which is the role of reconstruing or reinterpretation for therapists and clients. The importance of change to this approach is underlined. Not only is psychotherapy considered to be a continuing process, but the people participating in it are also seen as in process. The constructive alternativism so central to personal construct therapy is considered. I also deal with the abilities of therapists and clients to reconstrue because if we create our own constructs we can change them. Clients are victims, not of their pasts but of their interpretations of those pasts. Psychotherapy may be seen as, in essence, reconstruction. Also, because I have been dealing with the stories of clients and therapists, then therapy may be seen as the retelling of those stories.

THE IMPORTANCE OF CHANGE IN PERSONAL CONSTRUCT THERAPY

People are processes. Personal construct therapy values the subjectivity of people and such subjectivity is viewed as ever-changing internal processes (Bannister, 1970a; Rychlak, 1982). This account of people's experience has been extended to view people themselves as processes (Romanyshyn, 1982). People are continually changing (Goodman,

1978). This means that both clients and therapists are viewed as in process. For Frank, as a client, his internal processes were continually changing. He was in different phases of continuing conflict with his neighbors as well as with the shopkeeper he saw regularly. When he lacked such sources of stimulation of his anger, he found films with violence at which he could express it. When I tried to flow with these processes, I found Frank's anger very confronting. I therefore began my own process of making sense of his experience, with its attendant anger, as he shared it with me. Understanding his anger, in constructivist terms, should make my experience of it less confronting. I return shortly to the sense I made of it.

Psychotherapy is process too. Personal construct therapy, because it takes place between two people in process like Frank and me, is also process (Leitner, 1985). The processes of therapy are ever changing so that each therapy session will be different from the next (Barton, 1974; Goldfried, 1982). This view is apparent in other accounts of this therapy that describe processes such as anticipating, investing emotionally, and encountering, as well as confirming and disconfirming one's construing (Kelly, 1955, chap. 3 & 11). Christine's therapy with me was like this. We were both continually changing over our time together. For Christine, these changes fortunately involved movement from self-doubt to acceptance of her own abilities and from constricted, pessimistic construing to more dilated and even optimistic construing. For me, these changes included construing the changes in Christine. I was also modifying my view of the mutability of depression for people with Christine's courage to face some of her most distressing feelings.

CONSTRUCTIVE ALTERNATIVISM

Another constructivist assumption needs to be introduced at this point. The world, including the people in it, can be construed in a variety of ways (Kelly, 1955, chap. 3 & 11). Some of these constructions are better than others because they enable better anticipations of events. Yet, no one can yet construe a complete and accurate picture of the world so that approximations to that picture must be acceptable (Bannister, 1990b). All construing, then, as I indicated in Chapter 1, is likely to be either revised or replaced. There are always alternative construings available to people, and, therefore, to clients and therapists. This is the essence of *constructive alternativism.*

This important idea has direct and encouraging implications for clients who are feeling trapped by events or by their own construing, as Christine was. It also has implications for how people, and even mental health professionals, make sense of their worlds (Mischel, 1980). We may all be said to develop theories that vary from precise to elastic in their predictions. Psychologists need to have their theories, which underlie therapy, to reach a high level of precision; however, as people deal with daily events, their anticipations can be quite elastic. Theories, whether about the nature of the universe or of tomorrow's dinner, are patterns imposed by people on the changing events of life. These theories, however, being themselves events, can be construed on the basis of constructs from any other theory. Any theory can last only as long as these assumptions on which it is based continue to be accepted. Even the construing of formal theories like this personal construct theory of therapy, then, is subject to change. That follows from the assumption of constructive alternativism.

How alternative construing affects psychotherapy is now considered. All therapists and clients have theories that they test in psychotherapy (Mintz, Auerbach, Luborsky, Johnson, 1973). I began Frank's therapy with a general theory of how people change, something like that which I am proposing now. I also had a more specific set of suggestions arising from that theory about the extent of Frank's problem, which I initially saw as starting in construing which he had acquired at an early age and should not need to use now. He, too, had at least two levels of theories to do with his therapy. His more general theory was about how people change. Often it seemed that he saw great trauma as the chief source of personal change. He also had more specific suggestions from that theory about himself and his world. He saw his world as threatening to him and located most of the hostility that surrounded him in other people rather than himself.

Constructive alternativism is central to the therapeutic process because it permits alternative views of events to be considered and because both clients and therapists can choose to alter their views if they wish (Epting, 1984). This means that no theory of therapy, whether general or specific, can be final. Both clients and therapists are continually called on to change their theories. Frank and I were no exceptions. As I listened to his anger and the way it flared up when his control of his construing was threatened, I began to consider an alternative account of his problem. His description of his primitive treatment by his father during his childhood would have been sufficient to prompt the regression to constructs developed much earlier and reverted to during crises. However, there was other evidence as well, such as his better functioning with concrete actions than with abstract, verbal comments, to point to the possibility of more fragile psychological functioning. We together reconstrued these events of Frank's within and outside therapy and found that he had some unusual and very threatening beliefs about his world. He then came to regard himself as a person who needs to be careful to maintain control over his construing and to avoid situations in which that control is threatened. I describe more of how he came to this view shortly.

Theories of psychotherapy are alternative constructions. Theories of therapy may be applied either generally to predict how people change or more specifically about an individual client. Examples of both levels of theory application have been given from the therapies of Frank and Christine. All such theories provide alternative ways of looking at ourselves (Mahrer, 1992). They show how meanings interrelate or how constructs come together to enable construing to occur (Shainberg, 1980). They provide different ways of seeing the connections between events. They construct different frameworks for our storytelling. All our personal theories of ourselves and our worlds are merely alternatives to other theories, as are those shared theories which attempt to map the therapeutic processes (Mair, 1991). So is mine.

THE ABILITY TO RECONSTRUE

Creators of constructs can change them. People construe themselves and their worlds and then act according to their construing (Landfield & Epting, 1987). They do not react directly to the physical world but to their interpretations of it. Constructs, or personal meanings, are developed out of interactions of self and world. Worlds are structured by people imposing their own meanings on them. Fortunately, these created meanings are not applied so rigidly as to rule out choices between one construct and other, as constructive alternativism has shown. When interpretations are based on these created meanings, it is always possible to change them.

This ability of people to change their construing has formed the basis of some therapeutic work with people who are physically ill, who can be overwhelmed by anxiety, depression, and helplessness (Viney, 1991). When people become aware that they are responding to their construing of their illness rather than to that illness in its physical reality, they are no longer overwhelmed by the emotions generated by their construing (Viney, 1989). When they become aware of their own role in creating those constructs, they are well on the way to reconstruing. People coping with physical illness have been able, when they became aware of their ability to reconstrue, to change their construing from that laden with anxiety, depression, and helplessness to that associated with competence and other good feelings.

Clients need not be victims of their construing. For many decades, therapists' views of clients were influenced strongly by the psychoanalytic concept that people were the victims of their biographies (Freud, 1925). The traditional psychodynamic account has been that the experiences people have in their first 5 years of life will influence them markedly in later life. Personal construct therapy, however, offers an alternative view that clients are, rather, the victims of their own interpretations of their biographies (Kelly, 1955, chap. 3 & 11). I could even say that they are the victims of their autobiographies because they write these stories themselves. However, people can reconstrue the earlier events they remember throughout their life span. That reconstruing is limited by the permeability of the constructs used, that is, by the readiness with which my clients can apply them to make sense of new events.

Christine had, for some years, construed herself as the victim of that unfortunate assumption of her parents that she was pregnant:

Christine: I just couldn't go back to see them. What must they have been thinking of me! What must they think of me now! After all, my husband is the same man they disliked so much then. No, it's just impossible!

Yet, her recognition and expression of her fears of repeated rejection from them enabled her to entertain an alternative view of her relationship with her parents. This alternative was apparently available within her own construct system and had been temporarily suppressed by her fears of rejection. My contribution was to continue to accept her and her fears and not reject her, as she had expected. This disconfirmation of her construing of me seemed to trigger reconstruing of her relationship with her parents to the extent that she was not only able to go and stay with them, but also to use that time to make some new interpretations of herself and them:

Christine: I was really glad I went! I was able to talk with both Mum and Dad about some really important things. I asked Mum straight out how she felt about me when I was born, and she admitted that she had had a miscarriage just before me and was still a lot affected by that. It was good to know that I hadn't imagined her rejection attitude to me, and that we both understood it better.

PSYCHOTHERAPY AS RECONSTRUING

Reconstruing occurs in psychotherapy. The recognition of people's ability to reconstrue or reinterpret has been considered to be one of Kelly's (1955, chap. 3 & 11) most important contributions to psychotherapy. Of Kelly's followers, Fransella (1985, 1987) has been particularly aware of the importance of this ability in psychotherapy (Fransella & Dalton, 1990). She both defines therapy as requiring reconstruction and sees reconstruing as the essence of therapy. However, other personal construct therapists also consider reconstruing to be important. Constructive revision is required of clients (Viney, 1988), as well as changes in the content and organization of the constructs of clients which need to be assessed (Button, 1992). From a vantage point outside the constructivist approach, this type of therapy can be seen as awareness raising because it relies on both feedback and educational processes. This is in constrast with therapies that rely primarily on emotional catharsis or on the use of reinforcements.

Psychotherapy involves new construing. The constructivist approach sees therapists as having new theories of therapy available that emerge from old theories (Kelly, 1955, chap. 3 & 11). This is the transformative power of theory (Mair, 1991). Theories are, of course, special forms of stories that are particularly well integrated and created from construing, which is both permeable and abstract. Like all stories, they provide predictions. The theories of therapists shape what they do in therapy because it provides a framework for their stories. It also guides what they do to provide alternative frameworks for their clients. Rational emotive therapists (Dryden & Trower, 1988) also see this provision of new theories of living for clients as more important than their corrections of individual elements of irrational thought. However, I remind myself that it is not only my clients, but I as a therapist, who develop new theories during therapy.

PSYCHOTHERAPY AS THE TELLING OF STORIES

Psychotherapy is story-telling. Stories have been defined in personal construct therapy as filling a gap in our understanding of our own construing and that of others. They represent an integration of separate elements, here, as the narrative does in the study of literature (Mair, 1988b). Yet, the unit of integration is smaller than that provided by a whole system of constructs and larger than individual constructs; in fact, the story serves to integrate constructs or constructs and events. Both the content and the continuity of each story is put to the test, whether it be mine or that of my client (Viney, 1988). Such tests can be applied to the life stories of clients or to the more general psychological theories that have been seen to be the means by which we integrate what we know. The concept of the ongoing story should be particularly useful to this constructivist theory of psychotherapy because, as I noted at the beginning of this chapter, this therapy is about the processes of reconstruction.

Stories from the lives of clients and therapists are told in therapy. The stories that are woven into the therapeutic process are made up of other stories from clients and therapist (Cochran, 1986; Polster, 1987). Clients come to therapy with many stories that they have drawn from their lives (Hoshmand, 1993). Sometimes these stories can be grouped together under similar themes but sometimes a single one stands out that is more notable for its discontinuity with the others. These stories indicate how the clients construe themselves and their worlds. Clients also have some more general stories to tell about how they may change in therapy. Therapists, too, have these two types of stories about the client and more generally about change. These stories are influenced by the experiences of the people who tell them (Viney, 1994). This seems clear to me when my clients are involved but it is more difficult for me to recognize that my own formal theories of therapy are also stories that are much affected by my own life experiences.

Christine almost failed to start therapy with me because of the stories she brought with her from her life experiences:

Christine: If I keep on struggling on by myself, it will all turn out all right in the end.

Christine: When I admit to any weakness and ask for help, I'm rejected by the people I care about.

Christine: Life is terrible and I can't do anything about it.

These stories that Christine was repeating to herself were not shared with me initially. I had introduced myself to her as being concerned with her personal viewpoint, the stories she was telling herself, and the different levels of awareness she could have of these stories:

Linda: We are going to work together to understand your life better, and how you see it. This may be hard for you to do. The feelings you experience as we do this may well be painful. But the end result of our work here will be a bigger range of choices for you in terms of both feelings and actions.

Christine was able to respond to my stories of therapy in a way that made them relevant for her.

Storytelling is political. All stories are social. First, their content is often interpersonal (Viney, 1993). Indeed, the most important stories of psychotherapy are about relationships between self and others. Second, they are presented in a social context (Mair, 1988a). These stories are told by one person to another or to others (McAdams, 1985). The social content and context of therapy stories make them political, in other words, they have to do with power (Freiere, 1972). In their content, power can be ascribed in different ways. In the stories that therapists provide for their clients, they often indicate that much of the power is with them. The impact of such stories also varies according to their social context. Who tells them, to whom, and in what situation, as well as who controls their content, can also have political impact. Stories are, generally, powerful forms of knowledge and when a therapist tells a particular story to a client during psychotherapy, it takes on even greater power. Also, encouraging clients to tell their own stories can empower them.

PSYCHOTHERAPY AS STORY RECONSTRUCTION

Psychotherapy consists of the telling and retelling of stories. In therapy, clients and therapists tell their stories: therapists about therapy and clients about themselves and their worlds (Berger, 1989). The reconstruction or retelling of those stories begins. Both participants in therapy take part in these reconstructions so that therapy becomes the shared retelling of stories. Frank and I conducted such retelling. His original stories were as follows:

Frank: When I get confused, I get angry.
Frank: If I get angry, I could do a lot of damage.

My stories about Frank had developed as I saw more of him:

Linda: Frank does not handle frustration well.
Linda: He is easily confused, construes loosely and fears that he could lose control of himself.

We worked together to transform these stories about Frank into accounts of him that we could both accept as meaningful, integrated, and useful. The result was expressed, with some tightening from me, by Frank in this way:

Frank: If I let myself go, things could get out of hand. When I keep my anger under control, things are better. I can

> keep myself under control by taking it easy, exercising, keeping off the booze and doing what I enjoy doing. And I might need to see someone to talk about it all every couple of months.

We also decided that I would write a letter to Frank's physician in which I would tell him of our new accounts. Frank says that when he occasionally calls me for some support during a new crisis or to report an achievement of his that he keeps his copy of that letter handy and often rereads it.

Clients and therapists are tellers and retellers of stories (Viney, 1993). Clients are often the first to tell their tales, which are marked by sad and frustrated content and discontinuities, that I help them to reconstrue (Viney & Bousfield, 1993). Such reconstruction is not, of course, carried out without a close relationship between me and my clients. Often, clients are reticent about the stories that are really important to them until that close relationship has been established. They are also not always aware of the full story they have been telling themselves and they need help from therapists to make them explicit. Therapists, on the other hand, are responsible for making their stories that are relevant to the therapy sufficiently explicit for their clients to understand them. Therapists are also responsible for the stories their clients carry away with them about clients and therapists.

I was particularly concerned that Christine carry away with her after her six sessions of therapy stories about her therapist as a fellow human being and of herself as her own therapist. She had come sufficiently close to me to ascribe to me the rejecting role of her parents. The term *transference* is a label for her actions that is acceptable to constructivists (Kelly, 1955, chap. 3 & 11). It refers to a particular kind of story about oneself and others that is developed early in life and transferred to other people late in life without retesting its value as a predictor. I was at pains to ensure that Christine's transferred feelings for me were constrained at the end of therapy by a clearer view of who I am. In our last session of therapy, therefore, I made quite frequent references to my own life and feelings, about which I had been relatively silent earlier. Christine responded to this by starting to articulate a story about her own future more clearly:

Christine: I won't really need someone like you again, you know. If I get depressed, I know what to do. I'd stay around people this time, I won't avoid them. And I'd be able to see when I start getting in a rut and stop myself.

THE ROLE OF RECONSTRUCTION IN PERSONAL CONSTRUCT THERAPY

In the second and third sections of this book, I have examined the major assumptions of personal construct therapy. These are that people's meanings and purposes are important, although some are common to many people and others are unique to each one. Psychotherapy is a dialogue between two construers of meanings. The construings of therapists and clients are often best considered as stories that integrate a number of different meanings and so can be evaluated for both their content and their functions. In this chapter, I have dealt with my ability and that of my clients to recontrue. This constructivist idea results in a therapy that is about story reconstruction. In the next section of three chapters, I discuss in more detail the reconstructive processes of psychotherapy, beginning with goal setting and achievement and the therapeutic processes of reconstruction. Next follows an analysis of therapy as shared reconstruction.

READINGS

The Importance of Change in Personal Construct Therapy

Bannister, D. (1970a). Comment on H.J. Eysenck's explanation and the concept of personality. In R.T. Borger & F. Cioffi (Eds.), *Explanation in the behavioural sciences.* Cambridge: Cambridge University Press.*

Barton, A. (1974). *Three worlds of therapy: Freud, Jung and Rogers.* Palo Alto, CA: National Press Books.

Goldfried, M.R. (1982). *Converging themes in psychotherapy.* New York: Springer.

Goodman, N. (1978). *Ways of world making.* New York: Harvester.

Leitner, L.M. (1985). The terrors of cognition: On the experiential validity of personal construct theory. In D. Bannister (Ed.), *Issues and approaches in personal construct theory.* London: Academic.

Romanyshyn, R.D. (1982). *Psychological life: From science to metaphor.* Milton Keynes: The Open University.

Rychlak, J.F. (1982). Some therapeutic implications of logical phenomenology. *Psychotherapy, 19,* 259–265.

Constructive Alternativism

Bannister, D. (1970b). Science through the looking glass. In D. Bannister (Ed.), *Perspectives in personal construct theory.* London: Academic.

* Most useful readings.

Epting, F.R. (1984). *Personal construct counselling and psychotherapy.* New York: Wiley.
Kelly, G.A. (1955). *The psychology of personal constructs.* New York: Norton.*
Mahrer, A.R. (1992). *The integration of psychotherapies.* New York: Human Sciences.
Mair, J.M.M. (1991). Telling psychological tales. *International Journal of Personal Construct Psychology, 4,* 116–127.
Mintz, J., Auerbach, A.H., Luborsky, L., & Johnson, M. (1973). Patients', therapists' and observers' views of psychotherapy: A Rashomon experience or a reasonable consensus? *British Journal of Medical Psychology, 46,* 85–89.
Mischel, W. (1980). George Kelly's anticipation of psychology: A personal tribute. In M.J. Mahoney (Ed.), *Psychotherapy process.* New York: Plenum.
Shainberg, D. (1980). The relationship of theory to therapy. *Comprehensive Psychotherapy, 1,* 93–110.

The Ability to Reconstrue

Freud, S. (1925). *The collected papers of Sigmund Freud.* London: Hogarth.
Landfield, A.W., & Epting, F.L. (1987). *Personal construct psychology: Clinical and personality assessment.* New York: Human Sciences.
Viney, L.L. (1989). *Images of illness.* Melbourne, FL: Krieger.
Viney, L.L. (1991). A constructivist model of psychological reactions to illness and injury. In. G.J., & R.A. Neimeyer (Eds.), *Advances in personal construct psychology.* Greenwich, CT: JAI.

Psychotherapy as Reconstruing

Button, E. (1992). Eating disorders and personal constructs. In R.A. Neimeyer & G.J. Neimeyer (Eds.), *Advances in personal construct psychology.* Greenwich, CT: JAI.
Dryden, W., & Trower, P. (1988). *Developments in cognitive psychotherapy.* London: Sage.
Fransella, F. (1985). Individual psychotherapy. In E. Button (Ed.), *Personal construct theory and mental health.* Beckenham: Croom Helm.*
Fransella, F. (1987). Stuttering to fluency through reconstruction. In R.A. & G.J. Neimeyer (Eds.), *Personal construct therapy casebook.* New York: Springer.
Fransella, F., & Dalton, P. (1990). *Personal construct counselling in action.* London: Sage.
Viney, L.L. (1988). Psychotherapy as reconstruction. *International Journal of Personal Construct Psychology, 1,* 27–43.

Psychotherapy as the Telling of Stories

Cochran, L. (1986). *Portrait and story: Dramaturgical approaches to the study of the person.* Westport, CT: Greenwood.
Freiere, P. (1972). *Peadagogy of the oppressed.* London: Pergamon.

Hoshmand, L.T. (1993). The personal narrative in the communal construction of self and life issues. In G. Neimeyer (Ed.), *Constructivist assessment: A casebook*. New York: Sage.

Mair, J.M.M. (1988a). George Kelly, Don Bannister and a story-telling psychology. *International Journal of Personal Construct Psychology, 2,* 1–14.

Mair, J.M.M. (1988b). Psychology as story telling. *International Journal of Personal Construct Psychology, 1,* 125–137.*

McAdams, D.P. (1985). *Power, intimacy and the life story.* New York: Dorsey.

Polster, E. (1987). *Every person's life is worth a novel.* New York: Norton.

Viney, L.L. (1993). *Life stories: Personal construct therapy for the elderly.* Chichester: Wiley.

Viney, L.L. (1994). Reminiscence in psychotherapy with the elderly: Telling and retelling their stories. In B.K. Haight & J.D. Webster (Eds.), *The art and science of reminiscing.* New York: Taylor & Francis.

Psychotherapy as Story Reconstruction

Berger, I.W. (1989). Developing the story in psychotherapy. *American Journal of Psychotherapy, 43,* 248–289.

Viney, L.L., & Bousfield, L. (1993). AIDS and the client "in the fast lane": Narrative construction and reconstruction. *Psychotherapy Patient, 6,* 141–156.*

EXERCISES

1. Describe how both you, as a therapist, and your client can be said to be continually in the process of change.
2. What does the constructive assumption that all construing can be revised or replaced imply for you and your client in therapy?
3. Show how you and a client of yours have been able to reconstrue therapeutically together.
4. Has a client of yours needed to tell a story that he or she told in therapy? If you provided validation of the story did this prove to be therapeutic?
5. Describe a client of yours who was trapped by a story by which he or she lived. Were you able to retell these stories? If so, how?

IV

THE RECONSTRUCTIVE PROCESSES OF PSYCHOTHERAPY

7

The Goals of Personal Construct Therapy

In this chapter I present four sets of goals that I find are important to my clients and myself. The first set centers on awareness; that is, they include making meanings explicit, acknowledging the meaning of non-awareness, recognizing levels of awareness, and becoming aware of emotions, as well as of the power to reconstrue. The second set of goals consist of providing alternative stories for clients. These stories need not necessarily accurately reflect reality, although they may well. They must be viable narratives by which clients can live their lives. Clients also share our stories. All of those stories must be convincing to client and therapist alike. The third set of personal construct therapy goals involves clients in changing not only their construing, but also their actions in order to test the interpretations and predictions alternative stories make available to them. Such changes in their actions are related to changes in their construing, as an example of therapy with clients with relationship problems shows. When awareness, reconstruing, and changes in action patterns have been achieved by clients, it becomes possible to attain the last set of goals. These involve a choice of actions for clients, with alternative stories providing rationales for alternative courses of actions, and a view of their meanings as their choices about life. Yet, such therapeutic goals are not merely for clients. We therapists have our own goals to pursue during the therapeutic dialogue. Also, not all of the available paths for reconstruing are equally useful. This chapter therefore ends with a description of some criteria for selecting therapeutically valuable reconstructions from poor ones.

Before dealing with the major projects of personal construct therapy, however, I want to introduce two more clients of mine. Bob and

Ethel were also both sent to my university-based clinic. Bob was referred by his school psychologist at the age of 15 years old for "acting out," truancy, and inadequate school achievement. He was living at home with his father, mother, three younger brothers, and a sister. Although Bob was strong and healthy, his father had become unemployed as a result of disability brought about by multiple sclerosis. My other client, Ethel, at 83 years old, was at the other end of her life span. She was living alone. She was referred to me by her community health nurse because of my expertise in psychotherapy with the elderly. Her high levels of anxiety and social withdrawal were the main reasons for her referral. Although widowed, she was still living in her own home. She had one son and two daughters whose families lived nearby. Physically she was in good health but increasingly frail.

THE AWARENESS OF CLIENTS

Making meanings explicit is crucial to personal construct therapy. The first goal of personal construct therapists is to develop the awareness of their clients (Hobson, 1985). They help clients to make their often vaguely structured meanings more explicit (Barton, 1971). This implies that in the early stages of therapy the therapists are responsible for tapping into aspects of their construing of which clients may be unaware. As a therapist, I try to recognize their different levels of awareness of construing during therapy and, in the later stages of therapy, I work toward clients becoming more aware of their own abilities as construers and reconstruers. Bob's therapy with me shows how such a goal was agreed between us. When he came into my office for the first time, he was sullen and defensive. He was clearly frustrated by his long history of clashes with his school teachers and of failures to live up to their expectations. At that stage of our work together I had in mind the objective of him being able to articulate for himself what this meant to him. At that first interview, I also provisionally set the goal of having him explore the meanings of that other most significant event in his history as it had been reported to me, the deteriorating physical condition of his father and its implications for their respective family roles. There seemed to me to be a marked discrepancy between his performances as a reliable and dependable eldest son at home and his acting out at school. When I presented this discrepancy to him in our first therapy session, he was at a loss as to how to make sense of it. Understanding this discrepancy became a provisional goal I proposed myself for Bob initially but which we later contracted to work toward together.

The meaning of nonawareness for clients is also important for therapy. The construing of which clients are unaware is what therapists try to make explicit for them (Mahoney, 1988). These construings have been affecting their actions but remain beyond their awareness (Mahrer, 1986; May, 1969). In working to develop awareness of this construing, I sometimes try to experience for myself the events they are avoiding. To take another example, Ethel's anxiety suggested that she was finding that she could not make sense of what was happening to her by using her present range of constructs. Her community nurse had sensed anxiety in her and it was also apparent to me when I made the first of 10 home visits to her. She was pleasant and had thoughtfully arranged a cup of tea for me but there was an underlying tension in her manner that suggested continuing anxiety. When, in this session, we explored the meanings of various aspects of her life, she was able to provide coherent stories about her marriage, her motherhood, her contribution to the work force, and her widowhood. Her ability to provide integrated and meaningful stories about her life was in great contrast to Bob's inability, as befitted her greater psychosocial maturity. About two areas of her life, however, she was hesitant and constrained: her home and her adult children. As her therapist, I tried to experience what she was not able to tell me. There is more to report of those efforts later.

The *levels of awareness* of clients vary (Barton, 1974). Low levels of client awareness must be expected when their construing is expressed using meanings that are not readily shared by others or are not within the range of their own construct system (Kelly, 1955, chap. 3). Low levels of clients' awareness are also suspected when only one pole of their bipolar construct is accessible so that only one path of action is available to them. Such low levels of awareness can be suspected, too, or when the construct is suspended by other more important constructs in their construct system. Insight, in constructivist terms, requires being able to make sense of one's own actions (Kelly, 1955, chap. 3). Insight involves the effective use of constructs by people to interpret and predict their own actions. Clients can establish insight in therapy with only low levels of awareness but they cannot communicate it effectively either to themselves or to their therapists. So effective communication has become a goal across the range of constructivist therapies.

Awareness of their emotions is another integral part of personal construct therapy for clients (Kelly, 1955, chap. 3). Disruptive, negative emotions can easily become associated with their attempts to make sense of what happens to them and so block their effective use of their construct systems. This can be especially true for elderly clients who may have carried such disruptive guilt or fear of death through much of their lives. Ethel, for example, did not initially appear to be affected by either of these sources of anxiety but there was evidence of a low-level awareness in her construing of her relationship with her children. She showed it in the uniqueness of her constructs:

Ethel: I get on alright with them. They don't bother me, and I don't bother them. We paddle our own canoe.

She also showed it in her lack of an opposing pole for one of her constructs:

Linda: You mean you are independent of them, and they of you.
Ethel: Yes, and that works most of the time. But there could be a few things I can't do about the place.
Linda: When you say you feel independent of your family, what does that mean to you?
Ethel: It means I can do what I like when I want to.
Linda: And what about if you were not independent. What would life be like for you then?
Ethel: I don't know . . . it might be . . . Oh I don't know. See, I've never really been that way. My husband and me, we always did what we liked when we liked. When we ran the milk business, that's how we did it.

I was construing, by now, that one major source of anxiety for Ethel may be her inability to make sense of herself with the at least partial dependency required by her increasing physical frailty.

Clients need to become aware of their power to construe. Clients need to be able to share one of the most important ideas of personal construct therapy (Kelly, 1967; Mancuso, 1979). That is, they need to experience for themselves understanding themselves as construers and reconstruers. It is only when they, usually late in therapy, come to see themselves as having created their own meanings and as therefore capable of recreating new ones that I know that they have the power to leave therapy and continue with life, serving as their own therapists when necessary (Viney, Allwood, Stillson, & Walmsley, 1992). Bob was very far from this realization in the early stages of his therapy:

Bob: Things just keeps happening to me. The teachers pick on me. Some of the other kids have it in for me too. I seem to get sick a lot, you know. And none of that has anything to do with me. I can't help what happens.

Bob's construing was illustrative of the traps that such frustration and blaming of others can create for clients. He was cut off from his own ability to help himself.

ALTERNATIVE STORIES FOR CLIENTS

In this section, I deal with the viability of the stories of clients and their ability to make use of the stories their therapists provide. Yet, it is not only my clients who develop new stories, but also I as a therapist. It is the new stories of both clients and therapists that are shared by both participants in the therapy. Stories, it may be remembered, are narratives in which events and constructs are integrated. They provide order and purpose for the lives of the people who tell them.

Clients' stories need to be viable. Another goal of personal construct therapy is to supply new stories for clients, but not just any story is acceptable for this purpose (Sarbin, 1986). Acceptable narratives are not necessarily accurate but useful. Being useful means being easy to apply to events but at the same time providing different courses of action (White & Epson, 1990). They also should be convincing to both clients and therapists. Eventually, clients come to construct their own personal stories readily, independently, and securely. Bob was much in need of some stories in which he could have such confidence. His accounts of what happened to him at school, of which an example has been provided, were not viable. In particular, they were not providing him with suggestions for different actions he may try. Even Bob was only half convinced by his own stories and as his therapist I was not at all convinced by them. Another project that needed to be agreed with Bob was, then, the development of some different stories to account for his actions.

Clients come to share their stories. The power of the stories of therapists to transform the construing of clients often seems quite remarkable (Cox & Theilgaard, 1987). I find that clients can be easily influenced by the stories I tell, although not always in the directions I expected. There are many ways in which I can influence my clients and they can all contribute to the effects my stories produce. For example, Ethel's construing of her independence was often confused. However, as I listened to her account of it, I was reminded of that heroine of the Australian culture: "the little Aussie battler." The battler is typically a small woman looking after her family in either the town or the outback who works very hard physically to support the family but still finds the energy at the end of the day to provide her family with emotional support, albeit of a rough but caring kind. Ethel, having spent over 60 years construing herself in that culturally created and maintained way, had difficulty in developing any alternative view of herself. I resolved to work toward this project by sharing with her some of my stories of therapy with other elderly people. They had achieved a construing of themselves in which there is independence in some areas and some limited dependence in others.

Therapist, too, develop new stories. It is not only clients who reconstrue during therapy, but also therapists (White & Epson, 1990). In fact, psychotherapy is often successful only when both participants are able to develop new stories. When I first met with Ethel I concluded that because her anxiety relating to her possible dependence was paramount, anxiety about death was not a problem for her. I construed her as someone whose experience and understanding of dying was much more extensive than mine; this being another area of life in which I have as yet had relatively little experience. My construing in this area was also based on what I could see of her strong religious faith. However, before many sessions of therapy had passed, she challenged my story about her. Needless to say, this was somewhat anxiety arousing for me and prompted me to change my story:

Ethel: Yes, I've seen a lot of people close to me die. And people not so close to me too. But I still have this nagging doubt about passing on. I know I'll go to heaven, whatever that is like . . . and we can't know, so there's no point in worrying about it. But it's when I'm actually dying, I worry will there be someone there with me at the end? I often lie awake at night and think about that. I'd like to know there will be.

As well as recognizing her fear, I needed to revise my construing of her to take in one of her first expressions of some dependence on others.

These stories need validation. When one goal of personal construct therapy is to provide alternative stories for clients, an important criterion for their usefulness is whether clients and therapists can agree on them. This validation or confirmation by agreement is considered to be essential but there is still much debate between therapists about whose is the most important voice in this agreement. Those therapists who believe that therapists should take an open approach to therapy hear the client voice as dominant, whereas others believe that the professional voice (and construing) of therapists is at least as important (Rogers, 1959). I have noted that Bob's story about his actions at school did not meet my standards of usefulness. We therefore did not agree on an account of those actions and needed to create a shared account before we could progress further with his therapy. I suggested some different segments for his story:

Linda: I know you feel frustrated and angry at school, and that you think things at school make you feel like that. But are there other things, like at home, for example, that are frustrating for you?

Bob: No. Home's alright. I get on alright with the family, you know. It's just . . .

Linda: No times when you feel cross and cranky at home?

Bob: Well . . . sometimes, when I have to look after my brothers and sisters. . . . No. . . . But . . . that's alright.

It would be several sessions before Bob would entertain this change in his story.

CHANGES IN CLIENTS' ACTIONS

In personal construct therapy, changes in action are as important as changes in construing. Clients alter their actions when they test the viability of stories. When they alter the patterns of their actions they also alter their construing. I now provide an example of such changes in actions leading to changes in construing in clients with relationship problems.

Stories can be tested by action. Clients use their actions to test important questions about their stories (Bannister & Fransella, 1986; G.J. Neimeyer, 1987; Silberschaaz & Nathan, 1989. These are questions like: Does my story cover everything? Does it show what actions I can take? What happens when I try these actions out? It is only by proceeding in this way that clients can become their own therapists. When I came to confront his "I am not to blame" view of his problem, Bob needed to test out my revision of his story about his actions at school by being more cooperative, for example, at school and seeing how people responded to him then. Such a change in his actions was to be one of the goals we negotiated together eventually but only after much more reconstruing, the nature of which I report later.

Changes in action lead to changes in construing. Changes in the overt actions clients perform can lead to changes in their internal construing (Quattrone, 1985). Yet, a broader and more reflexive view of the relationship between them is that construing is action and action is construing (Epting, 1984). In other words, when people try to make sense of events their behavior is an integral part of this effect.

Whether I take the narrow or the broader view offered here, I believe that enactment of the problems of clients can be helpful to them in psychotherapy (Yablonsky, 1981). Enactment consists of acting out a set of problematic events in order to be able to reinterpret them. It can help to develop new courses of action. I deal more fully with its role in personal construct therapy in my next chapter. In the meantime, Ethel, like Bob, found that she needed to change some of her courses of action before she could feel comfortable in any kind of dependent role. Given that one of our shared goals came to be that she could be more dependent in certain areas if she wanted to be, Ethel also eventually set herself the more minor objective of letting her favorite daughter-in-law do some of her heavy cleaning. She would then work out what she could do for her daughter-in-law in return. This approach made a developing dependency more reciprocal and so more acceptable to Ethel's view of herself.

Action changes can be useful with relationship problems. One other powerful example of the effects on the construing of clients of their changes of action is worth reporting here. It deals with clients with problems in their relationships with other significant people in their lives. These clients have difficulty in understanding the construing of others (Bonney & Scott, 1983). It is difficult for them to put themselves in other people's shoes. They lack some of the shared construing that others have. They find it hard to grasp and act on the traditional roles of society, both their own and those of others (R.A. Neimeyer & Neimeyer, 1985). Whether they were treated individually or in group therapy for couples, enactment, or role play, taking on the perspective of others is an important part of what occurs for them. For example, they come to construe the inner worlds of others better and to share more construing with them. They also come to understand a range of societal roles better when they have been helped to reconstrue or reinterpret their own performance by observing how other people played those roles.

CLIENTS' CHOICES

The goals of clients include not only increased awareness, new stories, and changes in their actions, but also a range of choices of actions. These stories provide the rationales for the courses of action between which they choose. The meanings of their actions limit the choices they make about themselves and their worlds. *Stories serve as rationales for courses of action* (Ryle, 1992; Van den Berg, 1971). Alternative stories, then, serve as rationales for alternative courses of action. When, during therapy, clients come to consider different stories about themselves to be viable, they then have the necessary bases for different actions between which to choose (Fransella, 1985). That is why personal construct therapists ask, during their assessment of their clients, about the different courses of action they see as open. How aware clients are of their choices is also of concern. Ethel, it seemed to me, needed to develop alternative stories to enable her to acknowledge her ability to choose between being independent and dependent in day-to-day situations. Much of her anxiety was stemming from her awareness that her system of constructs was not enabling her to deal effectively with this area of her life.

Clients' meanings are their choices. For both therapists and clients, their meanings are their choices (Rychlak, 1982). This notion that it is their interpreting of events that limit their choice of action is a phenomenological and existensial one (Keen, 1977). The construing of clients has been arrived at by a series of choices and the less than fruitful choices they have made until now will continue to be made unless psychotherapy intervenes (Viney, Benjamin, & Preston, 1992). As a therapist, my aim is to enable my clients to live by choice and to be aware of doing so. Bob was living out a series of choices he had made about himself. He presently chose to see himself as the victim of a school environment that was hostile to him. The last of my therapeutic goals, then, was that he become aware of these choices and of the meaning of the contents of the story on which they were based. He was also to base these choices on a wider range of stories and to be aware of his own ability to choose his course of action.

SOME GOALS FOR THERAPISTS

As personal construct therapists, we have goals of our own to pursue during therapy. These goals or purposes we should make explicit to ourselves. They differ in their complexity. At the simplest level of construing, at the level of constructs, we have at least two goals that we try to achieve during therapy. We endeavor to make our constructs as permeable as possible; that is, we try to be open to using each construct to make sense of more and more events relating to our world (Kelly, 1955, chap. 3) and we also try to maintain our ability to use our imagination, to act as if rather than remain embedded in physical reality (Kelly, 1967). This human ability to construe as if, as well as "it is," is one of the constructivist assumptions I explored in Chapter 2. When I worked initially with Bob, both of these abilities were tested for me. My constructs about clients who will be able to make use of psychotherapy had some difficulty in making sense of his sullenness and resentment. For a time, this could have resulted in some sullenness and resentment of my own as I tried to validate my view of my world. The same aspects of Bob's initial reaction to me also challenged my ability to use my imagination effectively. Whether I was able to construe him as if he were potentially a reconstruing client would determine, to some extent, the outcomes of his therapy.

In order to understand clients effectively we need to have not only useful constructs, but also useful stories and construct systems. By "useful" I mean of value in interpretation and prediction. When we bring together a number of constructs to form a story, it must be structurally coherent and its contents must have some predictive value in terms of alternative courses of action in therapy. At the greatest level of complexity, our construct system must enable us to make sense of a wide range of events in therapy. Some of our goals in therapy are, then, to maintain and develop these aspects of our construing. With Ethel I had some difficulty in developing appropriate stories for and about her, partly because she had reached a phase in her own life span that I had not yet reached in mine (Lanfield, 1984). Many of the stories of my own 4th decade are about generativity, creativity, and helping others, whereas hers in her 8th decade are about an integrity of the many separate parts of herself, her life, and her world, which I can struggle to understand only partially (Viney et al., 1992). Ethel challenged a portion of my construct system. When this happened I first became aware of it through my own vague uneasiness. I then worked hard to develop that vague feeling until I could recognize it as an anxiety. However, acknowledging and identifying the sources of that anxiety, that is, those constructs of mine which were being challenged, enabled me to identify the aspect of therapy that was not being made sense of by using my available range of constructs. When Ethel's experiences became more meaningful to me in this way, my anxiety was greatly reduced. I was able to continue in effective therapy with her by continually monitoring my emotional reaction for my signs of that uneasiness.

SOME CONSTRAINTS ON RECONSTRUCTION

The major cluster of goals for clients in personal construct therapy deal with extending their awareness of themselves and their world, providing alternative stories for them, being aware of the alternative courses of actions offered by these stories, and using their abilities to choose between them. Goals for therapist, too, have been described.

Yet, reconstruction is not advocated by personal construct therapists for its own sake. Change for change's sake can have only limited value. Newer stories are not necessarily better ones. The stories developed by my clients and I during therapy must meet certain criteria.

Their content must be of general relevance to the experienced events and yet specific enough to make prediction possible. Their content must also suggest courses of action and be sufficiently optimistic about the outcomes of those actions to allow them to occur. The content of the stories of depressed people is often so pessimistic as to prevent action occurring. There are also criteria for the structure of our stories. Because they provide us with a way of organizing our construing, they must do this job well. They should also be well integrated with a whole story resulting that is greater than the sum of its construct parts. Stories should have an internal consistency, even a beauty, to them that is satisfying to client and therapist alike. By beauty, I mean personal appeal and "rightness." These criteria, then, are the means by which poor reconstructions are selected from good ones.

GOALS IN PSYCHOTHERAPY

In this chapter, I have discussed some of the most important goals of personal construct therapy. The first goal involves helping clients become more aware of their own meanings and the impacts of those meanings in their lives. The second goal involves providing alternative stories for clients. The third goal involves clients in changing their actions to fit with changes in their meanings and stories, whereas the fourth involves the wider range of choices for clients that result. We therapists also have goals to be aware of and achieve. In my next chapter, I show how this therapeutic process of reconstruing occurs.

READINGS

The Awareness of Clients

Barton, A. (1971). The client-centred transformation: A phenomenological approach. In A. Giorgi, W. Fischer, & R. Von Eckartsberg (Eds.), *Duquesne studies in phenomenological psychology* (Vol. 1). Pittsburgh: Duquesne University Press.

Barton, A. (1974). *Three worlds of therapy: Freud, Jung and Rogers.* Palo Alto, CA: National Press Books.

Hobson, R.F. (1985). *Forms of feeling.* London: Tavistock.

Kelly, G.A. (1955). *The psychology of personal constructs.* New York: Norton.

Kelly, G.A. (1967). A psychology of the optimal man. In A.H. Mahrer (Ed.), *The goals of psychotherapy*. New York: Appleton-Century-Crofts.*

Mahoney, M.J. (1988). Constructivist metatheory: Implications for psychotherapy. *Journal of Personal Construct Psychology, 1,* 299–316.

Mahrer, A.H. (1986). *Therapeutic experiencing*. New York: Norton.

Mancuso, J.C. (1979). Counselling from a personal construct perspective. *International Journal for the Advancement of Counselling, 110,* 305–313.

May, R. (Ed.). (1969). *Existensial psychology*. New York: Random House.

Silberschazz, G., Curtis, J.T., & Nathan, S. (1989). Using the patient's plan to assess progress in psychotherapy. *Psychotherapy, 26,* 40–46.

Viney, L.L. (1993). Goals in psychotherapy: Some reflections of a constructivist therapist. In L. Leitner & G. Dunnett (Eds.), *Critical issues in personal construct therapy*. Malabar, FL: Krieger.

Viney, L.L., Allwood, K., Stillson, L., & Walmsley, R. (1992). Personal construct therapy for clients who are HIV antibody positive. *Psychotherapy, 29,* 430–437.

Alternative Stories for Clients

Cox, M., & Theilgaard, A. (1987). *Mutative metaphors in psychotherapy*. London: Tavistock.

Rogers, C.R. (1959). A theory of therapy, personality and interpersonal relationships as developed in a client-centered framework. In S. Koch (Ed.), *Psychology: A study of a science*. New York: McGraw-Hill.

Sarbin, T. (Ed.). (1986). *Narrative psychology: The storied nature of human conduct*. New York: Praeger.

White, M., & Epson, D. (1990). *Narrative means to therapeutic ends*. London: Norton.

Changes in Clients' Actions

Bannister, D., & Fransella, F. (1986). *Inquiring man*. Beckenham: Croom Helm.

Bonney, W.C., & Scott, K.U. (1983). An explanation of the origin of role formation via psychodrama and personal construct theories. *Journal of Group Psychotherapy, Psychodrama and Sociometry, 36,* 46–55.

Epting, F.R. (1984). *Personal construct counselling and psychotherapy*. New York: Wiley.

Neimeyer, G.J. (1987). Personal construct assessment, strategy and technique. In R.A. Neimeyer & G.J. Neimeyer (Eds.), *Personal construct therapy casebook*. New York: Springer.*

Neimeyer, R.A., & Neimeyer, G.J. (1985). Disturbed relationships: A personal construct view. In E. Button (Ed.), *Personal construct theory and mental health*. Beckenham: Croom Helm.*

---

* Most useful readings.

Quattrone, G.A. (1985). On the congruity between internal states and actions. *Psychological Bulletin, 98,* 3–40.
Yablonsky, L. (1981). *Psychodrama.* New York: Gardner.

Clients' Choices

Fransella, F. (1985). Individual psychotherapy. In E. Button (Ed.), *Personal construct theory and mental health.* Beckenham: Croom Helm.
Keen, E. (1977). Existensial–phenomenological therapy. In D. Rimm & J.W. Somervill (Eds.), *Abnormal psychology.* New York: Academic.
Rychlak, J.F. (1982). Some therapeutic implications of logical phenomenology. *Psychotherapy, 19,* 259–265.*
Ryle, A. (1992). *A cognitive psychotherapy.* London: Sage.
Van den Berg, J.H. (1971). What is psychotherapy? *Humanitas, 7,* 321–370.
Viney, L.L., Benjamin, Y.N., & Preston, C. (1992). Personal construct therapy for the elderly. *International Journal of Cognitive Therapy, 4,* 26–35.

Some Goals for Therapists

Landfield, A.W. (1984). Personal construct psychology: A developmental perspective. *Journal of Social & Clinical Psychology, 2,* 97–107.*

EXERCISES

1. Select a client of yours for whom the goal of increased awareness of his or her construing is particularly important. Why is this so?
2. Select a client for whom the goal of establishing some alternative stories to his or her own is particularly important. Why is this so?
3. Select a client for whom the goal of a change in his or her pattern of action is particularly important. Why is this so?
4. Select a client for whom the goal of having a wider range of choices is particularly important. Why is this so?
5. Find a client of yours for whom reconstruction has been slow and difficult. What constraints have there been on this reconstruction?

8

The Retelling of Stories in Personal Construct Therapy

Story retelling in personal construct therapy can take many different forms. There are, first, certain basic processes of reconstruing that I examine in this chapter. They include the processes of validation and invalidation, loosening and tightening, and dilation and constriction, as well as the abstraction and concretization of my clients' construing. They can also involve becoming aware of constructs, changing the meaning of constructs, applying new constructs, and reorganizing entire construct systems. In story retelling, these basic reconstructive approaches are applied through a variety of therapeutic techniques, some of which I also discuss in this chapter. These techniques include a focus on the emotions of clients, the use of enactment or role play for which stories provide the plots, and avoiding story-based traps. They also involve using humor, interpreting dreams, and encouraging clients to develop and maintain meaningful relationships outside the therapeutic relationship. In this chapter, I write of the reconstruing of my clients, but such reconstructive processes are also available to me as a therapist.

In the previous chapter, I introduced two new clients who have worked with me and I explored in some detail the goals that we set for their therapies. It is their achievement of these goals that provide illustrations of the reconstructive processes and therapeutic techniques that I review. Bob, initially a sullen adolescent, had been referred for his acting out and poor academic achievement. His main therapeutic goals, which we now see fulfilled, were (a) a greater awareness of his construing of himself at school and at home, (b) viable but different stories for those areas of his construing, (c) new actions for those areas, and (d) new meaning-based choices. Ethel, an elderly woman, had been referred for her anxiety and social withdrawal. Her main goals were (a) greater awareness of her construing of herself and her family, (b) viable stories about her independence and dependence, (c) new actions for these areas, and (d) new choices about those actions. Also, both of these clients are seen to work toward that common goal for all personal construct therapy clients: greater awareness of self as construer and reconstruer.

THE BASIC PROCESSES OF STORY RETELLING

Validation and Invalidation

Two of the most basic processes of story reconstruction are validation and invalidation (McCoy, 1980) and they are especially important in psychotherapy (Fransella, 1985). *Validation* occurs when people's predictions of events are confirmed; *invalidation* occurs when they are not confirmed. People test their own construing for validity, usually through interactions with others. Personal construct therapists are an important source of validation for their clients (G.J. Neimeyer, 1987). Clients also may experience difficulties as they try to make sense of events that confirm or deny their construing. Therapists can help them deal with such difficulties. Yet, it is important for us to remember as personal construct therapists that not only do we have the power to validate, but also our clients. Clients confirm or deny our construing and our therapeutic techniques based on that construing. To return to our role as validator, we should also remember that when we invalidate the construing of clients, unless this is done very sensitively, the resulting interaction may be far from therapeutic. Such invalidation must be selective, focussing on problematic constructs which do not have a powerful influence on the clients' construct systems. Problematic constructs are those that do not provide clients with effective interpretation and prediction.

As Ethel talked with me during my weekly visits to her home, she often reminisced about events long gone. Such reminiscence in the elderly is considered to be evidence of a loss of sources of validation through bereavement (Viney, Benjamin, & Preston, 1988–1989). She had lost not only her husband and several children, but also many friends and other relatives. The main type of reminiscence was one in which she effectively wielded power. A brief extract from one of her reminiscences is provided:

Ethel: I used to have quite a say in what went on in this community, you know. I never joined any political party but I used to go to their meetings. They thought I didn't have much of a say, because I didn't speak up in the meetings; but I had my say with the other women afterwards when we were doing the washing up. And they had a big effect on who their husband voted for at the next election.

Many of these women who had confirmed Ethel's influence were now dead but she often repeated this kind of statement to provide herself with confirmation. As her therapist, I was able to validate some of this construing by encouraging her to talk about her influential role in her family even now. Later, I encouraged her to get her family to validate her construing in this area.

Loosening and Tightening

Loosening of construing in clients enables them to be more open to a wider range of interpretations (Epting, 1984). These interpretations can change easily but only to broadly related interpretations. It is achieved by techniques that are considered later, such as the analysis of dreams as well as those techniques which were as varied in their theoretical roots as free associations, relaxation, and genuine, respectful empathy for clients from therapists. When the construing of clients is loose, they can change the pole of the construct that they apply or even develop new frameworks for those constructs (Fransella, 1987). Although such changes are the essence of reconstruing, tightening is as important to psychotherapy as loosening for most clients (R.A. Neimeyer, 1986). *Tightening* of construing is characterized by the improved predictive power of clients' construing and its more effective and less changeable organization of constructs into stories (Epting, 1984). It is achieved by techniques reviewed in this chapter, such as enactment as well as by confrontation, and even by using the highly structured Role Construct Repertory Technique to help clients better understand how they are construing events. I encourage my clients to adjust to an appropriate balance between loose and tight construing. This is what I tried to do with Bob's as yet fragmented story about himself at school. His construing in that area was at first very tight:

Bob: All the teachers have it in for me. No way could I talk to them about what is happening, you know, none of them would listen to me.

When I introduced him to systematic relaxation and asked him to associate freely to the word *teacher,* he then loosened his construing considerably:

Bob: Teacher, preacher . . . see, they all tell you what you ought to do, you know. Teacher, friend . . . well, maybe some of them could be . . .

However, this construing was too loose for Bob's comfort and after some enactment of some classroom scenes, described later in the chapter, several sessions later he was able to achieve this balance between tight and loose construing:

Bob: I still don't like many of our teachers and wouldn't want to be one, but I guess they have a pretty hard time of it in the classroom. I think I can get on better with some of them now that I know that.

Dilation and Constriction

Both dilation and constriction of clients' construing are also important to their therapy (Kelly, 1955, chap. 7–8). Constructs, stories, and entire construct systems can all dilate and constrict. When they *dilate,* they broaden to deal with a wider range of events and this allows for some reorganization of construing. Clients whose construing is dilated are likely to see nearly all the events they experience as related to their problems. This ability can be useful but it can also lead to much confusion. *Constriction* of construing, in contrast, occurs when constructs, stories, or construct systems are narrowed to encompass a smaller range of events. Clients whose construing is constricted deal with only one issue at a time, which can also be useful for some phases of therapy but, if retained too long, interferes with taking a wider view as therapy draws to a close.

Neither dilation nor constriction alone is therapeutic, although clients sometimes use them together to achieve their therapeutic goals. I worked with Bob to dilate and constrict his construing of self at home in order that he could understand it better:

Linda: How does your father's illness make things different for you at home?

Bob: I don't know. . . . I guess I have to do more, like mowing the lawns and fixing the fuses when they blow. You know . . .

Bob was constricting his view of the impact of his father's illness on himself, so I tried to encourage him to dilate it a little:

Linda:	So you have some extra household chores to do now. And what about the other chores? Who looks after who in the family? Who do you try to help when they are angry or sad? And who helps you?
Bob:	Well, Mum gets pretty sad sometimes, you know. She cries a lot and that, but I leave that to my sisters. And I guess Dad gets sad too but he doesn't say anything. I mean, all I can do about that is get him to forget about it.

A clearer picture of Bob's view of himself at home was emerging, even if it still lacked his acknowledgment of his own sad and angry feelings.

Abstraction and Concretization

Constructs, stories, and construct systems can also be predominantly abstract or concrete (Kelly, 1955, chap. 7–8). Clients' construing becomes more *abstract* as it becomes more general and less related to the physical world and has a higher level of conceptualization. Such construing enables clients to understand the meanings of the complex and interrelated events in their lives. Their construing becomes *concrete* as it becomes more particular, more related to the physical world, and has a lower level of conceptualization. This construing enables them to understand some of their individual events and constructs. As for the earlier complementary types of construing, both of these types of construing have their role in therapy. Abstraction is the process encouraged by the assessment technique of laddering that is used to elicit the few superordinate or influential constructs. Concretization is used in pyramiding, by which clients come to understand better how particular constructs of theirs work in particular situations.

Laddering involves asking the question "why" of clients about a construct. After the preferred pole of his or her construct has been established, the client is then asked: "Why is this important to you?" The technique is called laddering because each consecutive "why" question asked taps into a higher, more abstract, and influential set of constructs. Bob, for example, spoke of the boys at his school as either "creepy" or, more rarely, "Okay to talk to" with quite concrete meanings assigned to the two poles of his construct. After he selected his preferred pole, I asked him: "Why are they Okay to talk to?" He replied: "Because they listen to you, not just look off in the distance." I continued the laddering by asking: "Why are they Okay for listening to you?" and he provided a more abstract construct contrasting "people who are open to others rather than closed." I continued to ask "why" about his preferred construct pole until we arrived at his superordinate and very influential construct: "People I like and people I don't." Pyramiding is used if a client needs to explore the concrete implications of mainly abstract construing. The questions asked then are "what" or "how," not "why." Pyramiding permits exploration of construing in the opposite direction from laddering toward the more concrete and numerous constructs.

Awareness of Constructs and Changing Their Meaning

Personal construct therapy can involve *becoming aware of construing*. Much of the construing that influences their actions people are unaware of. This does not lead to problems but just helps us to focus. This construing is described as preverbal. In some clients, however, lack of access to construing can limit their ability to reconstrue effectively. People who have dealt with trauma, for example, can lose their ability to talk about those traumatic events or even remember them. Natural disasters and more personal disasters such as rape can lead to such reactions. This dissociation can be part of a set of psychological problems described as Traumatic Stress Syndrome (Cromwell, Sewell, & Langelle, 1993). Crisis can have this effect too so that a reconstructive model of crisis intervention counseling involves helping clients to identify, acknowledge, and express their emotional reactions to the trauma, such as anxiety, depression, and anger (Viney, in press). The therapists working with this model try to understand the construing of their clients, verbalize some of their preverbal construing, including suspended constructs, and construct poles. They also further elaborate the construing of the clients and validate any of the clients' construing that provides the clients with more choices.

In therapy, *clients can change the meanings of their own constructs*, although this is not easy (Skene, 1973). Such changes can, of course, produce stories that are more coherent and useful to them. In a case of reconstructive therapy that I have described (Viney, 1981), the initial use of the Role Construct Repertory Technique showed Ethel to have very confused construing about her independence and dependence, but, by the time therapy finished, the Repertory Technique showed them to be much clearer and more viable.

Ethel's construing of her independence and dependence was also confused. She wanted passionately to remain independent with the meanings of that word that were important to her. One of those meanings proved to be that the relationships in which she felt independent were those in which she experienced some reciprocity:

Ethel: I feel comfortable with Junie (her granddaughter) when she helps out with the cleaning, because she doesn't mind me giving her children little gifts from around the house.

Linda: Do you also feel independent still with anyone else helping?

Ethel: Yes, there's the postie. He brings a few extra things up my hill for me, and I let him have some of my home-made wine for special occasions.

Linda: And how are these two relationships the same?

Ethel: We're both doing something for one another. I don't feel useless, like I do when some of the family help me. I feel useful.

Applying New Constructs and Reorganizing Construct Systems

Applying new constructs is even more difficult for clients to achieve than changing their meanings. Applying new constructs involves clients moving beyond their own meanings to use those of others (Viney, Benjamin, & Preston, 1988, 1990). It is for this reason that sharing of construing between clients and therapists is so vital to therapy. Clients often avoid developing certain constructs because they would, in applying them to themselves, find them in conflict with their own more influential construing. Sometimes it is these constructs that would provide them with more viable stories. Bob, for example, was initially resistant to any teacher-related constructs that recognized them as having a status similar to his own as a feeling human being. Although he could continue to view them as "the enemy" and "vermin," he could make them the target of the anger he apparently needed to express. It was when he started to explore such constructs of humanity with his friends and their parents that he began to explore more effectively the meanings for him of himself at school.

Reorganization of the construct system may also be necessary. If changing the meanings of old constructs and applying new ones is difficult for clients, then reorganizing constructs in their construct systems is even more so (R.A. Neimeyer & Harter, 1988; Viney et al., 1990). Yet, this is another means by which they can develop more viable stories. When clients have learned to view certain constructs as central to their construing of self, they cannot easily reduce their importance. Yet, to do so and replace them with other core constructs can open up many alternative paths for them. Bob showed this when he came to reorganize his construct system to see himself less often in terms of whether he was "victim" or "victor" and more often in terms of whether he was "follower" or "leader." He even came eventually to accept his own roles as construer and reconstruer:

Bob: I don't have to react when some of these teachers taunt me, do I? I can always decide I want to be the one who calls the shots, you know. And if I don't want to get into a battle with the teacher, I can always play it cool. I can see it the way I want to.

SOME TECHNIQUES THAT PROVIDE OPPORTUNITIES FOR THE STORY-RETELLING PROCESSES

A number of basic story processes have now been described. I have shown how clients can validate and invalidate, loosen and tighten, dilate and constrict, and abstract and concretize in therapy. I have also described and provided examples of how they can become more aware of their constructs, change the meanings of their existing constructs, apply new constructs, and reorganize some of the constructs in their construct systems. It is now time to examine some of the specific techniques that personal construct therapists use to promote therapeutic reconstruction. They invite clients to focus on their emotions, in order to accept and express them, and to use enactment in order to better understand their own construing and that of those close to them. Personal construct therapists also encourage clients to avoid choice-limiting traps in their construing and to share with them humor to remind them that alternative stories are available to them. Finally, they help clients to interpret their dreams and develop meaningful relationships to complement and later take over some of the functions of our therapeutic relationship.

Focusing on My Clients' Emotions

Emotions are central to personal construct therapy because intellect and emotion are inseparable in construing (Hobson, 1985). This statement holds for a range of constructivist therapies. Emotions occur as a result of whether clients' construing is validated or invalidated. As I said in the first chapter of this book, when validation occurs, positive feelings result; when invalidation occurs, negative feelings result. Feelings of guilt may occur, for example, if clients' core constructs about self are invalidated. Bob showed signs of avoiding recognition of such guilt feelings but his feelings of sadness proved more important.

When clients are not recognizing their own emotions like this, special techniques may be needed to foster awareness (Gendlin, 1981). Focusing on his bodily feelings and following them to his emotions worked well with Bob. He relaxed in his chair and, with my help, became aware of some of his bodily sensations. He reported a tightness in his chest that proved to be related to a similar constriction in his throat. He was able to identify this bodily message as sadness and then pursue what events in his life were linked with this sadness:

Bob:	I guess. . . . I don't know. . . . I guess it's Dad and Mum. I mean he looks so angry and hurt when he can't stand up by himself. And I don't know what to say to him. . . . You know. . .
Linda:	What would you like to say to him? Tell him now.
Bob:	I'm so sorry you're ill, and I wish I could do something about it.

Enactment

Enactment involves asking clients to act out an event on the basis of their construing in order to help them reconstrue it (Assogioli, 1973). I used it briefly in the previous excerpt in which I asked Bob to behave as if his father were present. The ability of clients to act as if, that is assumed by personal construct therapists, is the basis of the therapeutic use of enactment. If we want people to change, then we should treat them as if they were as we want them to be. Enactment can involve fixed-role therapy, role play, and psychodrama. The plots that clients enact represent their own and also a range of different stories. Therapists use enactment to open their clients to alternative views of themselves and their worlds, especially to the perspectives of the other people in those worlds. During these experiments, there is often evidence that new choices of action result from enactment.

The main personal construct therapy form of enactment is fixed-role therapy (Adams-Webster, 1981; Bonarius, 1970; Epting & Nazano, 1987). It requires clients to act out a standard role other than one of their own. That role is selected by clients and therapists together. The fixed role is created using clients' meanings; yet, these meanings are used somewhat differently from those clients' constructs in order that they do not slip accidentally between this therapeutic role and their own everyday role. The fixed role is selected so that it is relevant to the events with which clients are confronted and yet it extends their construing of them. It explores the implications of their old stories and develops new ones. It enables clients to experiment with their construing, first inside and then outside their therapeutic relationship. Many clients can benefit from acting out alternative roles they have with each of their parents, first with their therapists, then with friends and spouses, and finally, with the parents themselves.

The sadness, and even depression, that Bob shared with me seemed closely related to his anger at school. I therefore planned with him an enactment between himself and his teacher. His own role I defined in terms of his own initial self-construing and he played that role with me as the teacher as he saw him. We explored our reactions to that role play and then swapped our roles. This role reversal (Yablonsky, 1981) gave him a vivid picture of the possible construing, both intellectual and emotional, of his teachers and me a vivid picture of his construing. We then redrafted his student role to one construable using his constructs, but quite different from his former angry role, and based on his new understanding of the perspectives of his teachers. This he rehearsed with me with some success, which he appreciated more after another role reversal. Then he began to try out this new role of a more understanding and accepting student in the classroom. He did not lose his original story of his interaction with his teachers but filled it out until it was more coherent. He also found that his enactments had provided him with a range of alternative plots for that story.

Avoiding Story-Based Traps

Clients build *traps* for themselves out of their own construing (Viney et al., 1988). Often, their constructs come together to form stories, which trap clients into considering only certain kinds of actions to be available to them. This seems particularly common among elderly clients. One such client of mine, for example, had pulled two constructs together to form a story in this way: "I am a Scot" and "Scots are unforgiving." His resulting story ensured that he was maintaining some very frustrating, grudge-bearing relationships with his children as he grew older. Of course, they were using the same family story in their interactions with him. Personal construct family therapy was needed to enable them to change their self-defeating pattern of interaction.

Ethel's construing of herself as "the little Aussie battler" when linked into a story with another of her constructs "and little Aussie battlers are independent" provided a similar trap. The actions to which the implications of this story limited her were those that kept her living in a large house on her own and often refusing the help of her children because "I can do it myself." Ethel was, by her never-ending round of household and outside chores, missing some of the more relaxed entertainments of the elderly. She was actually depriving herself of her autonomy by trapping herself into continuous housework with her story about independence. How she came to work effectively on restructuring this story in therapy I have already described.

Using Humor

From a constructivist perspective, *humor* is very like metaphor (Viney, 1985). If people can interpret the major metaphors by which they live effectively, they can increase their control of their own lives (Mair, 1976). It is no wonder, then, that the explanation of clients' metaphors has been recommended in psychotherapy (Mills & Crowley, 1986; Witzum, Hart, & Friedman, 1989). The role of the metaphor in therapy as a provider of alternative stories has already been discussed. Like metaphor, humor involves clients and therapists in behaving as if. Therapists can use it to show how their clients' construing relates to the construing of others. It can provide a means by which their clients come to recognize their psychological problems. That is, when they, even in fun, acknowledge their own role as the construer of those problems, it saves them from the trap of naïve realism about them. Humor can also provide alternative stories for clients.

The use of humor in therapy, whether initiated by clients or therapists, has long been encouraged (Kuhlman, 1984; Saper, 1987; Viney, 1985). When therapists share humor with them, it can give clients alternative perspectives on their problems and a sense of control over them without oversimplifying those often complex problems. It can also provide a new representation of events for them that is helpful in itself; however, by its existence, it also increases their flexibility and opens them to the possibilities of change. Humor, in moderation, can also be used to establish or deepen a therapeutic relationship and to show respect for the client's view of the world, once that relationship has developed.

Some therapists may show a failure in the tact and sensitivity needed when introducing humor into therapy. When personal construct therapists introduce it, they try to be very sure that their construing remains within the range of their clients' construct system and that they are not stamping about carelessly in areas in which clients are experiencing distress from invalidation of their construing. I was careful to bear these constraints in mind as I was humorous with Ethel. She seemed to me to be likely to gain from it because she herself was humorous from time to time and had been happy to share that humor with me. "They used to call me 'Annie Get Your Gun' around here, 'cause I was so good with the rabbits. But now me legs and eyes have gone, it might as well be 'Annie, Get your Walking Stick.'" We exchanged a good deal of lighthearted banter like this to help Ethel understand more of her power as a construer. She eventually came to view herself as able to choose between different stories about herself and her world.

Interpreting Dreams

Interpreting dreams is a very important technique for personal construct therapists (Epting, 1984). Some therapists whose approaches are similar to constructivism even recommend that clients interpret their own dreams without the help of therapists (Gendlin, 1985; Gottschalk, 1985). I have been able to find relatively few descriptions in the therapy literature of personal construct dream interpretation. Dreams are useful to help clients become aware of events and their construing of events, of which they have been unaware (Kelly, 1955, chap. 7–8). Working with clients to understand their dreams on the basis of the assumption that all parts of dreams (all people and things) represent parts of their experience of which they are now aware can be helpful. Dreams may reflect a pole of a bipolar construct that has been suspended by clients. They may also represent preverbal construing that, because of its roots in the very early experiences of clients, has not been handled either cognitively or linguistically at the level at which those clients now function. Such dreams are often vague and contain no conversation. There are also "mile-post dreams" that, when dreamed by clients in therapy, indicate reconstruing by those clients.

Interpreting the dreams of clients provides them with opportunities for loosening their construing. It was this effect I was aiming for when I suggested to Bob that we interpret some of his dreams. He was initially a little suspicious about my motives and dubious about any useful outcomes. However, he enjoyed our joint attempts to make sense of his dreams and presented me with this one, which he said he had dreamed regularly since childhood.

Bob: I am lying somewhere, maybe on the bed, and I can feel myself very heavy. All my bones are heavy, like a skeleton's. This is very hard to say, you know . . . and there is this noise a really loud noise all around me. . . . It's the noise of a machine, you know, maybe like a lawn mower. It goes on and on.

Linda: Is that all? No feelings. No people or talking?

Bob: No, that's all. Just, a sort of, you know, uncomfortableness.

This dream bore no apparent relation to his problems at school. Neither did it appear to relate to his family interactions. However, it did have the vagueness, poor description, and lack of conversation characteristic of a dream representing preverbal construing. As we talked about it, it began to seem to me more and more like the experience of an infant in a cot isolated by machines. I suggested that he may have developed such construing if he was born prematurely and he rushed home to find out if he was. He had been 4 weeks premature, supported by machines, and physically cut off from his mother and father for 6 weeks after his birth. Such early events had laid the ground work for preverbal constructs that had later made it difficult for Bob to act according to his core role constructs as he perceived them both in the family and later at school.

Meaningful Relationships Outside Therapy

The other main technique of personal construct therapy involves ensuring that clients develop and maintain *meaningful relationships* other than their relationships with their therapists (Kelly, 1969). Dispersion of use of supports across many sources is favored clients over reliance on a small number of them. Some forms of constructivism has tended to focus more on the individual than on his or her social relationships, although this is of course not true of social constructionism. The importance of these continuing relationships for clients is that they provide sources, not only of support but also of validation of their clients' construing (Duck & Sants, 1983; Neimeyer & Neimeyer, 1983). Of course, friends and family in already established relationships with them may prefer to validate their old construing rather than their therapy-based reconstruing (Neimeyer & Neimeyer, 1985). It is for this reason that personal construct couple or family therapy may be necessary additions to individual therapy (Green & Kelly-Turner, 1990; Hoffman, 1992; Proctor, 1981).

I have found this to be so for elderly clients and their families and Ethel was no exception. When she started to accept more practical help from her sons and daughters, as a result of her reconstruing of independence, they were confused and even worried by these changes. Her son, Barry, said to me when he happened to meet me at his mother's home and she was busy: "She's a bit of a worry to us, you know. And now she's not even her old self. She was always so straight-backed and determined, I thought she's going to see me out." He was experiencing anxiety because his construing of his mother's strength was no longer being validated. Ethel, Barry, and I then decided to have a family council in which his mother's new wishes and roles in the family would be discussed. Five family members attended and they came fairly ready to understand not only the reasons for Ethel's new acceptance of their help, but also her interest in making that help reciprocal.

RETELLING STORIES: THERAPEUTIC STRATEGIES FOR CLIENTS AND THERAPISTS

Prospective clients of personal construct therapy can expect to experience certain kinds of therapeutic processes. First, they are likely to experience distress in the form of anxiety, depression, and anger. These emotions are the keys to invalidated construing. Clients also look at the available sources of confirmation of their construing among friends and family, as well as from themselves. Some validation comes from their therapists during therapy but they should not come to rely on them as long-term sources of validation.

Clients also come to expect to be invited to experiment with their construing in a number of ways. They may be asked to loosen or tighten their construing, broaden or narrow it, or make it more general or more specific. They may change the meanings of some of their constructs, substitute new ones, or reorganize their role in their construct systems. Such experimenting has as its objective the development of viable, alternative stories. The most important of these stories, which my clients select for use or not, is: "I have created my own meanings for myself and my world, and so I can change them if I choose."

In this chapter, I have shown some of the therapeutic processes of reconstruction but this has been largely from the perspective of clients. This presentation may sometimes have given the impression that these clients work almost alone but that is not so. Personal construct therapy takes place in a social context. In the next chapter, I talk about psychotherapy as reconstruction that is carried out jointly by clients and therapists.

READINGS

The Basic Processes of Story Retelling

Cromwell, R., Sewell, K., & Langelle, C. (1993, July). *The personal construction of trauma.* Paper presented at the meeting of the 10th International Personal Construct Congress, Townsville, Australia.

Epting, F.R. (1984). *Personal construct counselling and psychotherapy.* New York: Wiley.*
Fransella, F. (1985). Individual psychotherapy. In E. Button (Ed.), *Personal construct theory and mental health.* Beckenham: Croom Helm.
Fransella, F. (1987). Stuttering to fluency through reconstruction. In R.A. Neimeyer & G.J. Neimeyer (Eds.), *Personal construct therapy casebook.* New York: Springer.
Kelly, G.A. (1955). *The psychology of personal constructs.* New York: Norton.
McCoy, M. (1980). Positive and negative emotion: A personal construct theory interpretation. In H. Bonarius, R.S. Holland, & S. Rosenberg (Eds.), *Recent advances in the theory and practice of personal construct psychology.* London: Macmillan.
Neimeyer, G.J. (1987). Personal construct assessment, strategy and technique. In R.A. Neimeyer & G.J. Neimeyer (Eds.), *Personal construct therapy casebook.* New York: Springer.*
Neimeyer, R.A. (1986). Personal construct therapy. In W. Dryden & W.L. Golden (Eds.), *Cognitive-behavioural approaches to psychotherapy.* London: Harper & Row.
Neimeyer, R.A., & Harter, S. (1988). Facilitating individual change in personal construct therapy. In G. Dunnett (Ed.), *Personal construct psychology in clinical settings.* London: Routledge & Kegan Paul.
Skene, R.A. (1973). Construct shift in the treatment of a case of homosexuality. *British Journal of Medical Psychology, 46,* 287–288.
Viney, L.L. (1981). Experimenting with experience: A psychotherapeutic case study. *Psychotherapy, 18,* 271–78.
Viney, L.L. (in press). A constructivist model of crisis intervention counselling. *Journal of Constructivist Psychology.*
Viney, L.L., Benjamin, Y.N., & Preston, C. (1988). Family therapy for the elderly: A personal construct perspective. *Journal of Family Psychology, 2,* 39–48.
Viney, L.L., Benjamin, Y.N., & Preston, C. (1988–1989). Mourning and reminiscence: Parallel psychotherapeutic processes for the elderly. *International Journal for Ageing and Human Development, 18,* 237–249.
Viney, L.L., Benjamin, Y.N., & Preston, C. (1990). Personal construct therapy for the elderly. *International Journal of Cognitive Therapy, 4,* 211–224

Some Techniques That Provide Opportunities for the Story-Retelling Processes

Adams-Webber, J.R. (1981). Fixed role therapy. In R.L. Corsini (Ed.), *Handbook of innovative psychotherapies.* New York: Wiley.
Assogioli, R. (1973). *The act of will.* Baltimore: Penguin.
Bonarius, J.C.J. (1970). Fixed role therapy: A double paradox. *British Journal of Medical Psychology, 43,* 213–219.

* Most useful readings.

Duck, S., & Sants, H. (1983). On the origin of the species: Are interpersonal relationships really interpersonal states? *Journal of Social and Clinical Psychology, 1,* 27–41.

Epting, F.R., & Nazario, A. (1987). Designing a fixed role therapy: Issues, techniques and modifications. In R.A. Niemeyer & G.J. Niemeyer (Eds.), *A casebook in personal construct therapy.* New York: Springer.*

Gendlin, E.T. (1981). *Focussing.* New York: Bantam.

Gendlin, E.T. (1985). *Let your body interpret your dreams.* Wilmette, IL: Chiron.

Gottschalk. L.A. (1985). *How to understand and analyse your own dreams.* Berkeley, CA: Arts Reproduction Press.

Green, D., & Kelly-Turner, N. (1990). First steps in family therapy: A personal construct analysis. *Journal of Family Therapy, 12,* 231–250.

Hobson, R.F. (1985). *Forms of feeling.* London: Tavistock.

Hoffman, L. (1992). A reflexive stance for family therapy. In S. McNamee & K. Gergen (Eds.), *Therapy as a social construction.* Newbury Park, CA: Sage.

Kelly, G.A. (1969). In whom confide: On whom depend for what? In B. Maher (Ed.), *Clinical psychology and personality.* New York: Wiley.

Kuhlman, T.L. (1984). *Humour and psychotherapy.* Homewood: IL: Irwin.

Mair, J.M.M. (1976). Metaphors for living. *Nebraska Symposium on Motivation, 24,* 243–290.

Mills, J.C., & Crowley, R.J. (1986). *Therapeutic metaphors for children and the child within.* New York: Brunner/Mazel.

Neimeyer, R.A., & Neimeyer, G.J. (1983). Structural similarity in the acquaintance process. *Journal of Social and Clinical Psychology, 1,* 146–154.

Neimeyer, R.A., & Neimeyer, G.J. (1985). Disturbed relationships: A personal construct view. In E. Button (Ed.), *Personal construct theory and mental health.* Beckenham: Croom Helm.*

Proctor, H. (1981). Family construct psychology: An approach to understanding and treating families. In S. Walrond-Skinner (Ed.), *Developments in family therapy.* London: Routledge & Kegan Paul.

Saper, B. (1987). Humour as psychotherapy: Is it good or bad for the client? *Professional Psychology: Research and Practice, 18,* 360–367.

Viney, L.L. (1985). Humour as a therapeutic tool. In A. Landfield & F. Epting (Eds.), *Anticipating personal construct theory.* Lincoln: University of Nebraska Press.*

Witzum, E., Hart, O., & Friedman, B. (1989). The use of metaphors in psychotherapy. *Journal of Contemporary Psychotherapy, 18,* 270–290.

Yablonsky, L. (1981). *Psychodrama.* New York: Gardner.

EXERCISES

1. Use the technique of laddering to identify some of the most abstract and influential constructs in the construct system of a client of yours.

2. Help a dissociating client, who has been exposed to severe trauma, regain access to some of his or her lost construing. You should aid him or her to identify, acknowledge, and express his or her emotional distress, as well as reclaim his or her suspended construct poles.
3. Select a client of yours who has problematic relationships with his or her parents. Use role play, with role reversal, to work toward his or her taking on something of the parental perspective and trying out new ways of construing and acting.
4. Work with the dreams of a client of yours to tap into his or her preverbal or suspended construing.
5. Show how you have ensured, with a client of yours, that he or she has sources of validation for his or her useful construing of self from sources other than you.

9

Story Retelling Shared by Client and Therapist

In this chapter, I suggest that validation and invalidation of and by client and therapist are crucial to psychotherapy. Invalidation merits particular attention because although I may seek to invalidate the inappropriate construing of my clients, I must remember that they are often struggling with problems caused by continuing invalidation. Both clients and therapists make assumptions about therapy that influence how that therapy proceeds and they also have expectations about it that are similarly influential. These expectations involve ascribing specific meanings to each other because they are involved together in therapy. Examples of these expectations are provided, as are those for other expectations which may interfere with therapy. During the therapeutic sharing, clients and therapists influence each other. Some writers on therapy have considered that the therapist is the more influential but personal construct therapy assigns considerable power to both participants. This therapy is also seen as an interpersonal enterprise because clients and therapists are viewed as cotesters of stories. Such psychotherapy is, essentially, shared retelling of stories.

CLIENTS AND THERAPISTS AS MUTUAL VALIDATORS

Clients use their therapists as validators (Leitner, 1985). In other words, clients test and retest the effectiveness of their construct systems. Although some of this testing may eventually be with family and friends, much of it initially relies heavily on confirmation or disconfirmation from therapists. This means that personal construct therapists are careful to give as little unambiguous feedback to their clients as possible because in this tentative phases of their reconstruction they can easily misinterpret what is wanted. Validation is not, however, a one-way process (Bannister, 1975). The fact that therapists, and their therapy, are validated by their clients can be as important to therapists as validation of clients is to them. My own most central constructs, at this moment and for some time before, have been about whether I am useful or not. I can tolerate, I find, having some clients who do not confirm my view of myself as useful but I need to have some who provide evidence for this position.

Therapists do invalidate some of clients' construing. Their aim, in doing so, is to help clients to identify the inadequacies of their construct systems (Derlega & Berg, 1987; Soldz, 1988). This approach is somewhat similar to the cognitive-behavioral therapist's lack of reinforcement of the clients' assumptions that they judge to be inappropriate (Beck, 1967). It differs from the latter, however, in that it selectively involves subordinate and less infuential rather than superordinate and therefore more influential constructs. It is also always only an experiment carried out to try to help clients to understand their own construing better and not an attempt to direct their construing and actions into more acceptable paths. Such invalidation also differs in the awareness of a wider range of clients' construing than a cognitive-behavioral therapist would show that is necessary before such therapeutic experiments can be effective.

With 15-year-old Bob, I tried some invalidation of his construing of himself in several areas to enable him to see the limited courses of action they provided for him. One area was school in which he said of himself: "I am no good at this. I haven't the brains for it." When I acknowledged his continuing good work in the science laboratory, he was initially embarrassed but was soon able to extend his construing to include his successes. In the area of home, however, he had more difficulty. There he saw himself as, in contrast, "good. I don't rock the boat. I just do my chores and keep myself to myself." It took longer for him to recognize that this construing was preventing him from acknowledging and sharing his feelings of sadness with his family.

Some clients need to overcome continuing invalidation. There are clients who have had to cope with much invalidation or disconfirmation from their families (Kelly, 1969; Viney, Allwood, & Stillson, 1991) and I would not use further invalidation with them. They are sometimes diagnosed by professionals using other approaches as psychotic and their construing is thought to be so loose as a result of their experience continuing invalidation from others (Bannister, 1965). This account of psychotic construing is similar to that of the existential approach, which sees families as disconfirming the attempts by their psychotic member to develop a view of their world and, especially, to develop a sense of their own identity in relation to others (Collier, 1977).

Of the clients I have described here, neither Bob nor Ethel provide an example of this kind of process. Only Frank, of the clients who have agreed to contribute to this book, was sufficiently disturbed to do so. One of his stories showed that (during his early childhood but also into his teenage years) his father was both more demanding and punishing with Frank than he was with his other sons. Frank provided a vivid account of such invalidation in which his father, a pig farmer, often ordered him to clean out the pigstys after school. When Frank told him that he had finished, his father would claim that he had not done so and, in the face of the evidence of clean stys, make him start again claiming that they were dirty. Frank's mother and brothers never confirmed his construing that he had done the work, even though they saw him do so. With this information, it came as no surprise that Frank experienced much confusion and anger in later years.

CLIENTS AND THERAPISTS CONSTRUE EACH OTHER

During therapy, therapists and clients experience a mutual discovery of one another (Landfield, 1971; Viney, 1981). Therapists try to understand their clients' construing. In order to do so, therapists are as open as possible in their approach to them and follow their choice of language and metaphors. They also try to work with them as coevaluators of themselves and of therapy. Clients, on the other hand, have some similar processes operating in therapy, as I showed in Chapter 5. In their attempts to construe their therapists, they are, initially, both confused and anxious. They also tend, at least initially, to see their therapists as in control of what occurs. They usually do, however, try to understand their therapists' construing, as the therapists do theirs. As therapy continues, they come to see both as retellers of stories.

Ethel and I made many of these discoveries together. I tried to understand her construing of herself, for example, in relation to her family but at first found that to be difficult. This was probably because

I had not yet set aside my own current stories about family life with an elderly family member—my uncle whom I dwelled briefly on and later came to understand my own anxiety about his actions and then set aside issues regarding his having surrendered almost too much of his independence. When I became as open as I could manage, taking her view of the world as my own for a while, it became much clearer to me. Of course, I checked my understanding of her construing with her as my coevaluator as soon as I could. Ethel, for her part, was at first mystified about what I had to offer her, if I was not there to provide medical or housekeeping help. However, I do not think she was anxious because in her long life she could remember other mysterious events that turned out well. She tried to understand my construing of our therapy sessions and when she did so was able to see me as a reteller of stories and so a help in her development of new stories about herself as a construer.

THE THERAPY-RELATED EXPECTATIONS OF CLIENTS AND THERAPISTS

Special meanings of clients and therapists abound in therapy. Clients and therapists have specific expectations of one another, of which I give some examples (Hobson, 1985). Some clients whose expectations preclude shared reconstruction are examined. Before these aspects of the social context of therapy are discussed, however, it is important to note that clients and therapists assign special interpretations to each other because they are in therapy together (Mahoney, 1988). In other words, they attribute special meanings to each others' actions because their context is the therapeutic relationship. If they met elsewhere, even though their actions may be the same, they would interpret them differently. For example, Bob came to see me as different from the other adults he interacted with, such as teachers and parents, even though my actual words to him may at times have been the same as theirs:

Linda: Why do you think you've been behaving like that at school Bob?

Bob: You want me to tell how I was feeling then?

Linda: Yes.

Bob: Well, I was getting pretty angry and frustrated at home you know, and I didn't want to lay that on anyone there. So I guess I just let it out at school.

Linda: Umm. And how did that start?

Bob: I saw myself as no good at school and I couldn't see how I could be any different. It has helped to talk about this. I didn't think it would, you know, but I see things a bit differently now.

My questions in our last session together were questions any adult may have asked him but Bob interpreted them as having certain meanings within the context of therapy. As we developed more shared stories about what we were doing together in therapy, he was able to understand the intentions behind my actions from those stories.

Clients and therapists have expectations of each other. Indeed, much of the construing of therapists and clients consists of expectations about what each will do in therapy. Such expectations, of course, have implications for the actions of both participants (Bannister, 1983). Clients and therapists with similar expectations have been shown to have more complementary therapeutic relationships in which each acts differently from the other but in such a way that both sets of acts fit together (Benbenish & Schul, 1987). Those with different expectations have more symmetrical therapeutic relationships. These relationships can be seen as processes in which the shared reconstruing of expectations of each other has implications for the actions of both clients and therapists.

To provide an example of this reconstruing, I return to Ethel to show how her mystery of the visiting therapist was resolved:

Ethel: It's very nice of you to come and see me but . . . I don't want to be rude, but if you're not a nurse or a home help, then what do you do?

Linda: I help people sort out some of their other problems. Elderly people have a lot of other problems to deal with. Some of them are lonely. Some of them get worried about what is happening to them.

Ethel: Well, I'm not lonely. I've got more than enough family popping in and out of the house. But I do worry. I worry about whether the government will put up me pension soon, because things in the shops are getting more expensive every day.

Linda: You worry about whether you'll be able to buy food and clothes. Do you worry about other things?

Ethel: I worry about whether my body will see me out, and whether I 'll be able to go on like this.

Ethel was then able to negotiate with me very quickly a set of shared expectations about what we may do together, which were close to mine, and to act on them.

Some examples of matching client and therapist expectations are now provided. Several different pairs of matching client and therapist expectations have been identified. They can be defined largely in terms of the balance of power between clients and therapists but they also affect how the problems of clients are construed, the style of their interaction, and their actions. They not only affect the process of therapy, but also its outcomes (Collier, 1977). Metaphorically speaking, therapists and clients may act like doctor and patient, trainer and trainee, priest and penitent, friend and friend, or supervisor and researcher. All of these expectations are employed in some types of therapy (Pentony, 1981). The first three sets of expectations tend to place too much power with the therapist for me, whereas the fourth seems to deny the responsibilities of both therapists and clients to ensure that therapeutic processes are developed. The last of these, the notion of therapist and client as supervisor and researcher, is closest to my heart but it is too unusual a style of construing to be useful with most of my clients.

Some clients have expectations about therapists that do not permit them shared reconstruing. Personal construct therapy is based on the assumption that therapists and clients come to understand one another's construing (Kelly, 1955, chap. 12). For some clients, usually those diagnosed from other perspectives as psychotic, these role relationships will be too frightening and difficult (Leitner & Guthrie, 1993). The confusion of such clients enables them to avoid intimate relationships of this type (Leitner, 1988). In working with them, therapists need to take more of the initiative in developing such a relationship and proceed with caution. Anger is another way of avoiding these relationships. Confusion and anger remind me of my earlier client, Frank, whose psychological fragility I did not at first see for what it was. I came to recognize his avoidance of intimate relationships when I understood that his main sexual relationship had been for many years with a women who had married two different men during her relationship with him. When I began to understand the history of his construing of closeness, I suggested that our relationship continue as an occasional, supportive, telephone-based interaction, which it has. Had the extent of his anger been less, or had we been working in a hospital setting in which there was more support for both of us, I may have tried to establish a closer and so more effective therapeutic relationship with him; however, it would have been difficult.

THE INFLUENCE OF CLIENTS AND THERAPISTS

Therapists are initially seen as powerful. It seems to me that both clients and therapists have power in psychotherapy and there is extensive research literature that supports this assumption (Schwartz, Friedlander, & Tedeschi, 1986; Winefield, Bassett, Chandler, & Proske, 1987). Before this assumption is considered, however, it should be noted that many therapists who make nonconstructivist assumptions about their clients believe that therapists are much more powerful than clients (Pentony, 1981). In personal construct therapy, this view may hold only while the therapeutic relationship is developing. To find a client of mine who saw me as more powerful than he or she was, I had to go back to the other client in the first section of this book. Christine had difficulty in starting our therapeutic relationship because, depressed as she was, she felt both inadequate and vulnerable. She therefore construed any therapist who may work with her, who must of course be totally different from herself, as formidable and threatening. When, however, I continued to act with her in ways that were not so formidable or threatening, she was eventually able to apply different constructs to me as a potential partner in her reconstruing.

Clients and therapists are also mutual influencers. The constructivist view of the therapeutic relationship is that it is a two-way interaction: Clients influence therapists and therapists influence clients (Kelly, 1955, chap. 12). There is research-based evidence of these parallel attempts to influence (Friedlander, 1984; Friedlander & Schwartz, 1985; Tracey, Heck, & Lichtenberg, 1981). Both therapists and clients have been shown to direct their talk in order to manage the impressions each builds up of the other. These processes have been demonstrated in the 1:1 ratio of therapy, which is the focus of this volume, as well as in family therapy (Simon, 1988). The type of impression formed can of course determine the course of therapy. Clients who disclose their more personal material earlier are seen as more motivated and likely to succeed by their therapists.

This management of our impressions of each other was a form of influence that both Bob and I worked to exert. Although initially he was content to be seen as taciturn, he soon wanted me to view him more favorably. For my part, I wanted him to come to construe me as someone with whom he could share personal matters:

Linda: What important things have happened this week?
Bob: Well . . . I got on the football team. I'm pretty pleased about that. I'm not too bad at football you know.

Linda:	Who have you told about this?
Bob:	Not Mum and Dad, they're too busy. I wouldn't bother them with kids' stuff like that, you know.
Linda:	Umm. Do you have some friends you could tell how pleased you were?
Bob:	Yeah. I have one mate in particular. He was pretty chuffed for me! He's already on it.
Linda:	What is he like, I wonder?
Bob:	He's a good mate. You can really trust him, you know . . .
Linda:	If we could be mates like that for a while it would help you sort out a bit more what is going on for you.

CLIENTS AND THERAPISTS AS COTESTERS

The psychotherapeutic relationship has been described as being like a laboratory in which therapeutic testing can take place in the relative safety of this established relationship (Bannister, 1975). Clients and therapists can thus be viewed as cotesters who test the efficacy of the clients' construct systems. They do this both in the laboratory of therapy and the less safe environment of their interpersonal worlds. Clients explore with therapists their own construing and its implications for their actions. Ethel and I explored her construing of her independence in this way. Early in our interaction she was construing independence for herself so tightly that it prevented any acceptance of help from her family. Our explorations showed that, as a result, she was experiencing considerable distress, especially in the form of guilt. She was not meeting her own expectations for herself when one family brought a hot meal and another some fresh fish and she found them useful. It was only when our further explorations loosened her construing in this area that her anxiety began to decline.

CLIENTS AND THERAPISTS AS SHARERS OF STORIES

In psychotherapy, both clients and therapists tell stories (Gindhart, 1981; Polster, 1985; Zeig, 1983). Stories integrate and give purpose. The stories of therapists are primarily about the client in therapy and the world and those of clients are primarily about themselves in the world. The stories of clients often do not meet the standards needed to be useful for living their lives. For this purpose, they must be comprehensive and internally coherent to the degree appropriate to the events with which they deal. They also must be meaningful to other people and relevant for life. Ethel and I shared our stories, for example, about independence. Hers was as I have shown. I had a number of alternative stories, drawn from the professional and research literatures, the experiences of my psychotherapy team with other elderly clients, and my own experiences with my own elderly family members. In effect, I was offering her other comprehensive and coherent stories that other elderly people had found relevant for their lives. Two of these stories were: "Being physically dependent doesn't matter as much, so long as I am psychologically independent" and "I can enjoy having people do things for me and yet still feel useful and wanted."

PSYCHOTHERAPY AS SHARED-STORY RECONSTRUCTION

Psychotherapy is interpersonal process. I have argued that psychotherapy is process. This is in part so because it takes place between two people who are in process: the client and the therapist (Butler & Strupp, 1986). Yet, it is also because psychotherapy is always changing, with each new session being quite different from those before and after (Hobson, 1985). Psychotherapy also consists of communication, as an examination of the accounts I have given of the dialogues between my clients and myself shows.

Psychotherapy is also the shared retelling of stories. When therapists and clients start to share their stories, some of them may be changed (Fransella, 1985). Both clients and therapists take part in this retelling of the stories. In other words, the essence of personal construct therapy is shared-story reconstruction (Kelly, 1989). Such shared reconstruction results in shared stories in which therapist and client construing come to resemble each other. There is evidence that, as they work together, their expectations about therapy converge, as does their construing (Arizmendi, Beutler, Shanfield, Crago, & Hagaman, 1985; Benbenish & Schul, 1987). It also seems that similarity of values between therapists and clients is a good predictor of therapeutic outcome. What are values, if not stories, about how life should be lived?

Bob and I came to share many stories about how life should be lived. For example, I offered him the tried and tested therapist's story that, if he talked about his feelings more, he would be better able to deal with them. We modified this story, however, by adding that such expression may only occur if it was not upsetting to other people. This was because he still wanted to protect his parents from the full force of his anger.

RECONSTRUCTION IS INFLUENCED BY THE PSYCHOTHERAPEUTIC RELATIONSHIP

In this chapter, I have described personal construct therapy as shared reconstruction. Such reconstruction is influenced by the therapeutic relationship. Because therapeutic reconstruction takes place in a social context, the outcomes of that reconstruction are at least in part determined by the interpersonal factors that are at work. This is apparent in the way in which the retold stories that emerge from therapy are influenced by validation and invalidation by both my clients and I. It is true that I sometimes use invalidation of my clients' construing which seems to me self-defeating or limiting. Yet, clients also exert control over this process because past responses to their construing may result in them not considering certain stories of mine to be acceptable. What reconstrued stories emerge from therapy is also influenced by the stories my clients and I develop about each other and about therapy. Our expectations also influence the stories we develop and they can prevent clients from the intimate sharing that is the essence of psychotherapy.

The stories that are selected for retelling are also a function of the therapeutic relationship because both clients and therapists influence each other during therapy. We also work as cotesters; in other words, we share this active role. We share stories and so the stories that emerge eventually are influenced by those that have been contributed. Stories from my clients come from their personal experiences, whereas mine come from my personal experiences but are developed, too, from the experiences I have shared through therapy with other clients and my professional and literary reading. We reconstrue stories together and as we do we share more of our construing. It is on this recognition of the importance of shared reconstruction that my most often used individual personal construct therapy strategies, described in the next chapter, are based.

READINGS

Clients and Therapists as Mutual Validators

Bannister, D. (1965). The genesis of schizophrenic thought disorder: Retest of the serial invalidation hypothesis. *British Journal of Psychiatry, 11*, 377–382.

Bannister, D. (1975). Personal construct theory psychotherapy. In D. Bannister (Ed.), *Issues and approaches in the psychological therapies.* London: Wiley.

Beck, A.T. (1967). *Depression: Clinical, experimental and theoretical aspects.* New York: Harper & Row.

Collier, A. (1977). *The philosophy and politics of psychotherapy.* Sussex: Harvester.

Derlega, V.J., & Berg, J.H. (Eds.). (1987). *Self-disclosure: Theory, research and therapy.* New York: Plenum.

Kelly, G.A. (1969). In whom confide: On whom depend for what? In B. Maher (Ed.), *Clinical psychology and personality.* New York: Wiley.

Leitner, L.M. (1985). Interview methodologies for construct elicitation: Searching for the core. In F. Epting & A.W. Landfield (Eds.), *Anticipating personal construct psychology.* Lincoln: University of Nebraska Press.

Soldz, S. (1988). Constructivist tendencies in recent psychoanalysis. *International Journal of Personal Construct Psychology, 1,* 329–348.

Viney, L.L., Allwood, K., & Stillson, L. (1991). Reconstructive group therapy for HIV seropositive patients. *Counselling Psychology Quarterly, 4,* 243–254.

Clients and Therapists Construe Each Other

Landfield, A.W. (1971). *Personal construct systems in psychotherapy.* Chicago: Rand McNally.

Viney, L.L. (1981). Experimenting with experience: A psychotherapeutic case study. *Psychotherapy, 18,* 271–278.

Therapy-Related Expectations of Clients and Therapists

Bannister, D. (1983). The internal politics of psychotherapy. In D. Pilgrim (Ed.), *Psychology and psychotherapy.* London: Routledge & Kegan Paul.*

Benbenish, R., & Schul, Y. (1987). Client–therapist congruence of expectations over the course of therapy. *British Journal of Clinical Psychology, 26,* 17–24.

Hobson, R.F. (1985). *Forms of feeling.* London: Tavistock.*

Kelly, G.A. (1955). *The psychology of personal constructs.* New York: Norton.

Leitner, L.M. (1988). Terror, risk and reverence: Experiential personal construct psychotherapy. *International Journal of Personal Construct Psychology, 1,* 251–262.*

Leitner, L., & Guthrie, A.J. (1993). Validation of therapist interventions in psychotherapy: Clarity, ambiguity and subjectivity. *International Journal of Personal Construct Psychology, 6,* 281–294.*

Mahoney, M.J. (1988). Constructivist metatheory: II. Implications for psychotherapy. *International Journal of Personal Construct Psychology, 1,* 299–316.

---

* Most useful readings.

Pentony, P. (1981). *Models of influence in psychotherapy.* London: Collier Macmillan.

The Influence of Clients and Therapists

Friedlander, M.L. (1984). Psychotherapy talk as social control. *Psychotherapy, 41,* 335–341.

Friedlander, M.L., & Schwartz, G.S. (1985). Toward a theory of strategic self-presentation in counselling and psychotherapy. *Journal of Counselling Psychology, 32,* 483–501.

Schwartz, G.S., Friedlander, M.L., & Tedeschi, J.T. (1986). Effects of clients' attributional explanations and reasons for seeking help on counsellors' impressions. *Journal of Counselling Psychology, 33,* 90–93.

Simon, R. (1988, September–October). The constructivist challenge: An interview with Lyn Hoffman. *Networker,* pp. 55–59.

Tracey, T.J., Heck, E.J., & Lichtenberg, J.W. (1981). Role expectations and symmetrical/complementary therapeutic relationships. *Psychotherapy, 18,* 338–344.

Winefield, H.R., Bassett, D.L., Chandler, M., & Proske, I. (1987). Process in psychotherapy as decreasing asymmetry between patient and therapist: Evidence from the verbal interaction. *American Journal of Psychotherapy, 41,* 117–126.

Clients and Therapists as Sharers of Stories

Gindhart, L.R. (1981). The use of a metaphoric story in therapy: A case report. *American Journal of Clinical Hypnosis, 23,* 202–206.

Polster, E. (1985). Escape from the present: Transitions and story line. In J. Zeig (Ed.), *The evaluation of psychotherapy.* New York: Brunner/Mazel.

Zeig, J. (1983). Erickson's use of anecdotes. In J. Zeig (Ed.), *A teaching seminar with Milton Erickson M.D.* New York: Brunner/Mazel.

Psychotherapy as Shared-Story Reconstruction

Arizmendi, T.G., Beutler, L.E., Shanfield, S.B., Crago, M., & Hagaman, R. (1985). Client–therapist value similarity and psychotherapy outcome: A microscopic analysis. *Psychotherapy, 22,* 16–21.

Butler, S., & Strupp, H. (1986). Specific and nonspecific factors in psychotherapy: A problematic paradigm for psychotherapy research. *Psychotherapy, 23,* 30–40.

Fransella, F. (1985). Individual psychotherapy. In E. Button (Ed.), *Personal construct theory and mental health.* Beckenham: Croom Helm.*

Kelly, G.A. (1989). *The function of interpretation in psychotherapy: Techniques of psychotherapeutic reinterpretation.* London: The Centre for Personal Construct Psychology.

EXERCISES

1. Show how, during therapy, you and a client of yours served as validators of one another's construing. What kind of constructs were validated for the two of you?
2. Listen to some tapes of a set of therapy sessions with at least two of your clients. How does the power balance in your relationship change within and between sessions? Between clients?
3. Plan with a client of yours some therapeutic tests for the two of you to carry out, first within your therapy sessions and then in his or her interpersonal world. When you try them, how successful are they? How could they be improved?
4. What stories have you and your clients shared? To achieve what therapeutic goals?
5. Have some of your most effective therapy been with clients who shared some of your values? What values? Have some of your least effective been with clients who did not?

V

STRATEGIES FOR PERSONAL CONSTRUCT THERAPY

10

Some Therapeutic Strategies for Individual Clients

This chapter is concerned with the strategies used during therapy with individual clients. In the next chapter, I focus on strategies used with groups of clients. Therapists, especially those in training, often have concerns about how to begin therapy. I start with that, focusing on what they do in the first session to make sense for clients of the roles of client and therapist, and their therapeutic relationship. They also work to build up generally therapeutic expectations in their clients. Therapists then need to be able to understand their clients' construing as quickly as they can but they also need to monitor it, with them, throughout therapy. The strategies employed then include listening to clients and using a range of constructivist assessment techniques. There are also some freer and more imaginative techniques for clients and therapists to use together while clients tell stories that are central to their construing.

Then there are the therapeutic strategies used to help clients in the retelling of their stories. These involve sharing the analysis of their construing and enactment of problematic aspects of it. They also embrace all the many techniques that can be used to help clients test the predictive power of their construing. There are also the strategies that aid clients in taking a perspective on their own construing, seeing themselves as construers who have the power to change their own construing if they choose. The last of these strategies are those which promote the retelling of stories. This chapter concludes with some comments on the ending of therapy, a most important and also difficult aspect of the therapeutic process. Here I focus on how therapists help their clients to make sense of their own role after therapy, the new role of the therapist, and their future relationship together, underlining their sense of personal power.

BEGINNING THERAPY

Making sense of the clients' role is where personal construct therapy begins. Clients need, at the beginning of therapy, to have some useful ways of understanding not only the therapist role and the therapist–client relationship, but also their own role as clients (Button, 1985). They will have some expectations about these roles but they will not necessarily help them to work effectively in therapy or fit with those of the therapists (Viney, Benjamin, & Preston, 1992). Of course, therapists need to know what those expectations are. They may ask some of their clients: "What do you think you will do when we work together?" However, other clients do not, at that stage of their possibly first interaction with a therapist, articulate their dim notions and vague fears. Therapists may also ask some clients: "Why are you here? What do you hope to get from these sessions?" Of course, showing clients how the therapist answers questions like these can also be helpful so that with some clients they may explain briefly how they came to be there and what they expect will happen when they work together, but that is likely to come later in the first session. Asking clients if they have any questions can also be useful in allowing them to raise issues that are very important to them that therapists have ignored. The most common method, however, is to ask them a general question like: "How are things for you at the moment?" and then to listen to their response. Some depressed and withdrawn clients do not pour out answers to such a question but then to share some silence with them even at this stage of therapy can be a very companionable and encouraging experience.

There are also three other aspects of their role that can be raised with clients during that first session of therapy. The first of these is that the choice of whether to come to the therapy session or not is theirs. Personal construct therapists believe that that must genuinely be the case. This is, after all, their first indication that clients have the power to make choices. If therapists try to work with clients for whom attendance at sessions is compulsory (e.g., in schools, prisons, or psychiatric hospitals), they may be unlikely to draw power from the interactions. The second of these aspects of the client role is that clients may experience emotional distress, as well as a wide range of good feelings, during therapy. This is because the central process of this form of therapy is reconstruction, or reinterpretation, and any such change in people's ways of making sense of their world is associated with distressing emotion. The third aspect has to do with the central role of the client in personal construct therapy. For example, the therapist may tell clients: "What happens in these sessions and what you get out of them depends a lot on you. If you put a lot of yourself into them, you'll get a lot out."

Making sense of the therapists' role is crucial to beginning therapy also. Clients also have expectations about how therapists will act (Epting & Boger, 1981). Again, the obvious and often useful way to find out what they are is to ask them: "What do you want from me in these sessions? What do you think I can do for you?" Therapists need, of course, to give their clients some notions of how they see their own role. The essential ingredients of this role are those prized by most therapists. They need to be seen as accepted by clients, honest with them, and listening carefully to their stories with some ability to think and feel about them as they do. (No, I don't always achieve these parts of my role with all clients on all occasions. However, I explore the possible sources of blocks to these achievements, both in personal reflection and in peer supervision.) I find that there is often little to be gained by talking to clients about these aspects of the role but that I can communicate them best by "doing" them. And this doing starts before my clients arrive for their first session in the way I arrange the room we work in before they come. It is also apparent later when they can see the time I take (or try to) between sessions to reflect on what they have been telling me.

The therapeutic relationship needs to be understood. Learning how to be comfortable together is one of the first tasks of clients and therapists at the start of therapy. Only after that aspect of the therapeutic relationship is established will they be able to work together effectively (Fransella, 1972). Establishing the confidentiality of the relationship can aid in this process, as can explaining some aspects of the therapeutic process. Monitoring of the clients' ways of making sense of the world is, for example, the task of not only therapists but also clients. Another example has to do with the interaction of the two roles in therapy. Clients work and therapists help. A third example concerns the role of questions in personal construct therapy. Therapists ask a lot of questions, clients ask a lot of them, and sometimes therapeutic progress can be identified not through their finding of answers but through the finding of better questions. Clients need to know that they will not always be able to answer the questions of the therapists, and neither will the therapists. Of course, apparent in this initial construing of the therapeutic relationship are many explicit contracts between therapists and clients. However, it is at the end of that first session that a more explicit contract between them is usually drawn up about how long the therapy will be, where and when, and what goals (perhaps only preliminary ones at this stage) they plan to achieve.

Building therapeutic expectations is also important. The initial therapy session is also the time to start to build some general expectations for clients that should, the therapy literature shows (Dunnett, 1985; Viney, Allwood, Stillson, & Walmsley, 1992), lead to effective therapy. Therapists try to convey hope that the goals they have considered together will be achieved and confidence that client and therapist have the ability to do this. This hope and confidence is probably conveyed more in the way things are said than what is said. Showing them how they can be more powerful as a result of this time together is also important. This can be difficult because many clients feel quite powerless during their first session and believe that they neither have the ability nor the right to make those kinds of choices. Again, that they do have this power can be demonstrated to them at this early stage by emphasizing the choices available to them then, such as when and how often they come for therapy sessions.

UNDERSTANDING CLIENTS' CONSTRUING DURING THERAPY

The main strategies used to help therapists understand some of their clients' construing during therapy can be classified into four groups: (a) listening to constructs they use as they talk; (b) employing techniques from other personal construct therapists; (c) employing even freer, more imaginative techniques; and (d) listening to their stories and telling some of their own. I have already provided examples of the use of these strategies in earlier chapters of this book.

Listening for the constructs that clients use can be done in at least three ways. The simplest of these is attending to the words they choose to use (and using the same words), checking that the meanings coincide. Therapists also listen to their choice of metaphors. Some clients express themselves readily in metaphor, whereas others do not. However, even those who do not refer to them often have a life metaphor that guides their actions and this can be an important key to their construing (White & Epson, 1990). Therapists also listen for their clients' expression of negative emotion either directly or indirectly (in their tone of voice and posture). Such emotion provides clues to what parts of their construct systems are not operating effectively. With anxiety, identifying the area of their lives in which events are occurring that are beyond the range of their constructs is useful. With anger, searching for the area or areas in which they are continuing to use constructs that are no longer receiving validation is more so.

These listening strategies have been for therapists to use. There is, however, a form of that listening (for constructs, metaphors, and distressing emotions) that can be shared by clients and therapists. If they agree to tape their sessions, then clients and therapists can play them back to jointly identify their most important construing and its implications for their actions. This procedure is useful only for selected segments of some therapy sessions and only with some clients. It is most effective with clients who tend to avoid reflecting on their own experience and actions and need the distance provided by listening to the recording to enable them to do so.

Therapists have developed a number of useful *constructivist techniques for understanding construing*. These techniques are laddering and pyramiding, the Repertory Grid Technique, self-characterization (Chapter 8), and what has come to be known as, rather mysteriously, the ABC Model. Laddering and pyramiding have been described already (Chapter 8). *The Repertory Grid Technique* involves an increasingly structured series of steps, not all of which need to be taken (Bannister & Mair, 1966). It provides information not only about the content of clients' constructs, but also how they relate to one another and how they are applied to important people and events (Beail, 1985). When interpersonal relationships are of interest, the important people in clients' lives are compared, three at a time, in such a way as to provide descriptions of both poles of a bipolar construct. I may ask: "Think of your mother, your father, and your sister. How are two of them alike and one of them different?" A client may reply: "My mother and sister are warm and easy to be with but my father is so irritable and cross." This basic comparison can be used as part of the ongoing therapeutic interchange as well. It provides a useful way of establishing both poles of the constructs of clients. The full Repertory Grid, the grid of ratings of important people construct by construct, is often used only when therapists are still at a loss about the content and interrelationships of their clients' construct systems or, later in therapy, if they are still at a loss themselves.

Self-characterization and the ABC Model remain to be considered. *Self-characterization* involves asking clients to write a character sketch of themselves as if they were a character in a play (Fransella, 1981). They are asked to write about themselves from the outside like this so as to be threatened as little as possible. There is no right or wrong way for them to do this but therapists try to leave them as free as possible to decide how long, for example, it should be. This can be particularly useful relatively early in therapy because it helps therapists begin to see their world through their clients' eyes. Their first sentence often gives a vivid picture of how they see themselves, whereas the body of the self-characterization can provide information about the areas of reconstruing that are most likely to occur.

The *ABC Model* provides information about the areas of construing in which change is least likely to occur. This is used later in therapy if clients seem to be blocked in their attempts to change. It enables them to explore the implications of moving from one pole of a construct to its opposite pole when construing themselves (Dunnett, 1988). *A* refers to this construct, with *A1* being the pole presently in use and *A2* the opposite pole. *B1* and *C2* represent the disadvantages of each pole and *B2* and *C1* represent the advantages. An example from a client seems necessary here. Sally was a 17-year-old who felt that she wanted to stop smoking, yet every attempt by her to do so failed. The ABC Model of her construct of herself as a smoker or nonsmoker proved to be as follows:

A1	Smoker	A2	Nonsmoker
B1	Poor, not much money; parents have a go at me	B2	Better of financially; get my parents off my back
C1	Relaxed, feel grown up	C2	Get pretty churned up; everyone'll think I'm just a kid

It is no wonder that she had not been able to stop smoking because it not only made her feel better, but also was seen by her as an integral part of becoming an adult.

There are also some even *more imaginative techniques* that can be used by both clients and therapists for understanding the construing of clients (Dalton & Dunnett, 1993; Leitner, 1985). Drawing or painting can be used in place of the highly verbal techniques I have been describing. A simple curved line can be presented to clients on a piece of paper and they can be asked to continue the line to draw the construct they are having difficulty expressing in words. This difficulty can be because threat has attacked their verbal capacities or because those constructs have always been preverbal. Of course, clients need to use language eventually to communicate effectively with their therapists and probably with themselves too; however, this initially nonverbal technique can often help them move past a verbal barrier. Both therapists and clients come to understand more of the clients construing when their drawings, and what they represent to them, are discussed (Thompson, 1989). The same benefits can come from using other media beside pencils or crayons and paper, for example, Plasticine or clay modeling of a construct or the writing of a piece of music about it. The encouragement to use a little imagination can be liberating to clients. Yet, there are also times when imagination can be useful to therapists. Therapists can learn while listening to their clients' accounts of their thoughts and feelings to develop images that prove to express the most central constructs of those clients. Such images are often visual but they can be auditory or conceptual. This capacity comes readily to some therapists but, I must admit, not to me.

Storytelling by clients and therapists is another helpful strategy for understanding the construing of clients. However, the most important job in coming to understand the construing of clients is still not done if some of their most influential stories have not been identified (White & Epson, 1990). To have the scraps of information about clients' construct systems, provided by this knowledge of some of their constructs and how they are applying them to individual events in their lives, is not enough. Therapists need to know how they bring them together to make up the stories that influence their lives. Both the content and form of those stories are considered. Their content needs to include predictions about the outcomes of action that are precise enough to choose an appropriate action and optimistic enough to make it possible. Their form should be well integrated and internally consistent. It is when these criteria are not met that therapists start to look at how they may be retold and even bring in some stories of their own to help with that reconstruction.

HELPING CLIENTS TO RETELL THEIR STORIES

The therapeutic strategies that are used in personal construct therapy to achieve its therapeutic goals are almost infinite in their variety. I see them as falling into five categories. The first of these categories involves analysis of their construing, a breaking down of it into identifiable parts. The second of these involves enactment, in which clients actually do what their constructs prompt them to do. The third includes strategies that primarily enable clients to test the predictive value of their constructs, whereas the fourth involves them in taking a more distant perspective on their own construing. All of these types of therapeutic strategies contribute to and often precede the major strategy of helping clients to retell their stories. This is the fifth type of therapeutic strategy I discuss.

Analysis of Clients' Construing and Enactment

All of the strategies that result in further *analysis of clients' construing* lead to new construing that is tighter rather than looser, constricted rather than dilated, and, generally, concrete rather than abstract, although there are exceptions to this (Kelly, 1955). Their new construing involves precise and unchanging narrowly focused and reality-based interpretations of events. One of these strategies, which is an exception, is that which involves therapists helping clients to identify significant events and people in their lives and identifying and expanding their construing of them. Another such strategy, with more specific outcomes, is that of helping clients to describe their own constructs. When this is done with pencil and paper it is a particularly effective technique for tightening construing. Yet another analytic strategy that tightens focuses on clients' purposes, intentions, and goals. Therapists and clients compare the current status of clients with their aspirations and hopes, whether those projects are validated by others, and by whom and in what circumstances.

Enactment is an even more powerful reconstructive tool. It consists of doing, not just talking. This involves clients and therapists in recreating significant events so that the construing, and especially the emotions clients have associated with it, can be experienced more fully, tested, and placed properly in the context of relationships with other people (Kelly, 1955). Enactment generally results in clients loosening their construing, so that it has more possible outcomes, and dilating it, so that it makes sense of more events. However, it also has concretizing effects, bringing emotionally detached clients to the realities of the situations in which they live and work. Enactment is a particularly powerful strategy for reconstruction because of the very close relationship between people's construing and their actions that influence each other and are, in turn, influenced. It is also a useful tool when clients cannot find the words to express themselves effectively (Jennings, 1987).

Enactment can be used in a number of ways. It usually begins within therapy sessions but it can continue into the everyday world. It also begins with the simple acting out of aspects of clients' views of themselves or of events that have been significant for them but it can continue into the playing of complex dramas involving several people and perspectives (Yablonsky, 1981). In such dramas, reversal of role between clients and those whom they see as reacting problematically to them can be very useful in enabling them to see events from other perspectives. It is from these different perspectives that the choices about how my clients can construe the world come.

Fixed-role therapy (Epting & Nazario, 1987), a form of enactment developed by personal construct therapists, has already been mentioned. To begin, it involves asking clients to write a self-characterization. An example from Sarah, written in the third person as if by a friend, follows. Its constructs are underlined:

> She is a mother and wife with a wonderful family. She is a hard worker, and puts a lot of effort into her family.
> She also puts a lot of effort, into her home which is beautifully looked after.
> She is not a confident person, though, especially about being with others. She is shy and finds it hard to get to know others. She does not like to go to parties or even have the neighbours in for a barbeque.

A role for them to act is then developed using their constructs as much as possible rather than those of the therapists. This role is, in part, similar to clients' views of themselves but it is also in part drawn up so that it goes some way to achieving their goals for them. A role to permit Sarah to experiment with socializing can be described in this way:

> This other woman that you will play is Madge, who is a mother and wife who puts a lot of effort into her home and family. She is confident when she meets people outside her family and enjoys being with them.

When an appropriate role has been worked out between therapists and clients, clients then start to act as though they were that person with some of those achieved attributes. Usually the playing of the fixed role begins in situations that they feel are not so important for them so they are free to find out what happens when they take the risk of acting differently. Later playing of the role then occurs in more important and potentially stressful situations. The value of this type of enactment lies in the way it works within the constraints of clients' construct systems but allows them to test the effects of changes in some of their most inflexible construing. This can be very difficult for them and continuing support and validation from therapists is very important to them at this time.

Testing Construing

Of all the strategies that help clients to retell their stories, those that enable them to *test their construing* are among the most basic. Clients cannot decide that retold stories are better for them unless they are getting feedback about the effects of those stories on their relationships in the first place with their therapists but also with the people in their everyday world. All therapeutic strategies provide such testing of predictive power to some extent. For example, enactment does so. They do not have to be therapeutic techniques based primarily on a constructivist psychology to be useful for this purpose. All the therapeutic techniques that therapists are currently familiar can be used to enable clients to test the efficacy of their construing, regardless of the theoretical assumptions from which they were developed.

A brief reminder of some of those techniques seems useful here, together with some available readings about them at the end of this chapter. They also serve to loosen or tighten clients' construing, dilate or constrict it, and make it more abstract or concrete. In fact, these techniques can be grouped roughly according to their effects on these forms of clients' construing. The first set is one of therapeutic techniques that loosen and dilate the construing of clients and cause it to become more abstract. Their new construing involves changeable, broadly focussed, and generalizable interpretations of events. These techniques include the free association (Freud, 1925) and dream analysis (Gottschalk, 1985) of the psychoanalytic therapists, meditation (Blows & Srinivasan, 1991), the "empty chair" technique of the gestalt therapists (Fagan & Shepherd, 1971), and art therapy (Dalley & Case, 1992; Rubin, 1987). The second set of categories creates a different kind of construing altogether. They lead primarily to client construing that is more tight, constricted, and concrete. They include cognitive restructuring, reframing, goal setting, and other cognitive-behavioral techniques for dealing with anxiety, depression, and anger (Beck, Rush, Shaw, & Emery, 1979; Rudestam, 1980), the homework and contracting of behavior therapy (Kendall, 1985), some techniques from rational-emotive therapy (Ellis, 1979), and transactional analysis (Berne, 1964). Transactional analysis provides a metaphorical language with which clients can construe more effectively their interpersonal interactions.

The third and fourth groups of therapeutic techniques have only single differences from the two sets I have already described. One of these loosens and dilates clients' construing, like the initial group, but lead to it being more concrete rather than abstract. The strategies in this group are psychodrama (Yablonsky, 1981) and the body therapies (Mahrer, 1986), the focusing of the existential therapist (Gendlin, 1981), and relaxation training (Wolpe, 1969). The latter can be seen, for example, as loosening clients' construing of their anxiety, dilating their construing of anxiety-related events, but concretizing their actions in response to that anxiety. The other set of therapeutic strategies tightens and concretizes construing but dilates it as well. One such specific technique is assertiveness training (Rudestam, 1980). All of these techniques from other therapeutic approaches provide opportunities for clients to test their construing in a way that is central to personal construct therapy.

Taking a New Perspective on Construing and Story Retelling

Taking *a new perspective on their own construing* is something personal construct therapists encourage all of their clients to do. The particular perspective in focus is that of recognizing themselves as construers and reconstruers and as creators and recreators of their own meanings (Fransella, 1981; Viney, 1989). This also involves seeing themselves as having the power to recreate their view of their world and to retell their stories. This is, of course, a constructivist perspective. It offers them some distance from their problems and the thoughts and feelings about them and it also, as a result, offers them a choice of actions (Worden, 1991). When small children become lost in a maze it is fun for a while but can become frightening and overwhelming; yet, when they come out and view the maze from a hill above it, the maze again seems to them fun and not at all threatening. Much the same is true of life's problems. Taking this new perspective can be achieved by clients experiencing it in therapy, by therapist example, and by humor. It can loosen or tighten, dilate or constrict, or abstract or concretize the construing of clients. The actual effects depends very much on how their construing was at the beginning of therapy.

It is the *retelling of stories,* especially those of clients, that are crucial to personal construct therapy (Viney, 1988). For some clients, such retelling involves me in identifying gaps in their story line. For others, the focus is on showing that there is an integrated, construct story line that they have not seen. This integration may be over time so that they develop a sense of their own history and development or it may be over events so that they can see the consistencies of their reactions from situation to situation. For yet other clients, encouraging them to search their memory for alternative stories to compare with their current stories, either personal or family stories, can be helpful (Crose, 1990; Webster & Cappeliez, 1993). Others can benefit from the stories therapists have to tell, either personal stories or those from their training as therapists. Others make use of stories from a wider variety of sources, such as a bibliotherapy sourcebook (Rubin, 1978). Clients use all these sources of stories when they come to select a story or stories about themselves to retell so that it provides them with some choices in their courses of action and sufficient optimism about them to make acting on them worthwhile.

ENDING THERAPY

It is appropriate to be concluding this chapter on what to do as a personal construct therapist with a few words on how to end therapy (Landfield & Epting, 1987). There is much to do at this time and much of it is difficult for clients and therapist alike because it requires much reconstruing. There is also so much that is new to make sense of: the changed role of the client, the changed role of the therapist, and how their relationship is to continue. Encouraging a sense of power in clients as therapy formally ends is also important. I say formally because in one important sense, personal construct therapy never ends because clients continue as their own therapists.

Making sense of the new role for clients is central to the ending of personal construct therapy. I find it is very important to arrange the ending of therapy so that my clients are often reminded of when it will recur. This is true whether 5 or 25 sessions have been planned. Direct verbal statements about it are useful but so are a host of less direct reminders that therapists can give. Clients need to notice, for example, changes in the content of our concluding discussions. They become broader in their focus, being encouraged to even veer occasionally into casual conversation. Therapists can also begin to underline with them the good things in their lives, their sources of enjoyment, as well as their own strengths. This can help to maintain, in understandably anxious clients, that sense of optimism necessary for them to continue as their own therapists.

Making sense of the new therapists' role is another important aspect of ending therapy. The therapists' role changes in many ways at this time. There are several tasks for which therapists become responsible. One is to be human and to be occasionally superhuman to reduce any transference that may have developed. Another is to encourage clients to continue to monitor their own construing and actions so that if they judge that they need further therapy then they can set out to find it. The other two tasks have to do with the responsibility of therapists to monitor their own actions and their implications for other people (Pilgrim, 1983). The first involves securing from clients an evaluation of the successes and failures of therapy as it has gone so far. The second involves working on similar evaluations of it with professional colleagues who do not know the identity of the clients. This consultation with people outside the therapeutic relationship can be very helpful, especially just before the last session or two with clients, so that therapists review, as clients review for themselves, what has happened.

Making sense of the new therapeutic relationship is also central to ending therapy. Although the decision not to continue with therapy sessions has been made, this does not mean that is the end of the relationship between clients and therapists. Clients and therapists now have stories that incorporate the other that they will consult from time to time. Neither does this decision mean that they can have no more contact. Therapists like to know how they are faring and some clients like to know that their therapist is available if they need support or encouragement. With most clients, therapists make sure they know how to contact them in the future, usually by giving them the telephone number on which they have a reliable and confidential answering machine if not available. With me, they seem to ring as often to report their ups as their downs. With more fragile clients, I tend to arrange some forms of regular ongoing review, for example, so that they make, say, first a monthly and then a bimonthly report. Some therapists use a standard 3-month follow-up letter to all their clients. This seems especially useful in the anonymity of a large service in a large city.

There is one other change in the therapeutic relationship that takes place as therapy ends, on which I want to comment. This relationship between clients and therapists has been an unusual relationship in many ways. In particular, they have been in a very close and intimate relationship (Epting, 1984) and yet they have probably touched one another very little. It seems to me appropriate, then, to mark these good-byes by some brief touching that is meaningful to both. What form this touching takes is going to vary with the styles of individual clients and therapists. My own vary from the simple but expressive handshake, to a friendly punch on the arm at one extreme, to the full, frontal bear hug on the other.

Just as it was important for clients to begin therapy with expectations that would help with therapy, it is now important that *clients leave therapy with a sense of their own power* (Bannister, 1983). This will help them to cope better with many events in store for them but will also enable them to continue as their own therapists when therapy finishes. Therapists try to make sure that their clients are aware, therefore, of all the skills they have learned during therapy. They also have developed considerably more understanding of themselves and probably of other people too and they can apply this knowledge as their own therapists. They have also developed the ability to take a constructivist perspective on their problems, one which acknowledges their role in creating their own construing and actions and their ability to choose others. Above all, they now have a fund of stories, about themselves and others, on which they can rely for strength and for the knowledge that they have the power to choose their course in life. To have some written stories of this kind to take with them from therapy can be helpful (White & Epson, 1990).

DOING RECONSTRUCTIVE THERAPY: SOME STRATEGIES

In this chapter, I have tried to deal with some of the practical implications for myself as a personal construct therapist. I have considered what I find myself doing as therapy begins and ends. Yet, between those topics I have also described what I do in order to understand my clients' construing during therapy and how I help them to retell their stories. I dealed with some of the strategies I use for both assessment and psychotherapy with individual clients. In the next chapter, I consider some of the therapeutic strategies used with groups of clients.

READINGS

Beginning Therapy

Button, E. (Ed.). (1985). *Personal construct theory and mental health*. London: Croom Helm.

Dunnett, G. (1985). Construing control in theory and therapy. In D. Bannister (Ed.), *Issues and approaches in personal construct theory*. London: Academic.

Epting, F.R., & Boger, P.A. (1981). Personal construct psychotherapy. In R.L. Corsini (Ed.), *Handbook of innovative psychotherapies*. New York: Wiley.*

Fransella, F. (1972). *Personal change and reconstruction: Research and treatment of stuttering*. London: Academic.

Viney, L.L., Allwood, K., Stillson, L., & Walmsley, R. (1992). Caring for the carers: A note on counselling for the wider impact of AIDS. *Journal of Counselling and Psychological Development, 70*, 441–446.

Viney, L.L., Benjamin, Y.N., & Preston, C. (1992). Personal construct therapy for the elderly. *International Journal of Cognitive Therapy, 4*, 26–35.

Understanding Clients' Construing During Therapy

Bannister, F., & Mair, M. (1966). *The evaluation of personal constructs*. London: Academic.*

* Most useful readings.

Beail, N. (Ed.). (1985). *Repertory grid technique in personal construct: Applications in clinical and educational settings*. London: Croom Helm.
Dalton, P., & Dunnett, G. (1993). *Living with personal construct psychology.* Chichester: Wiley.
Dunnett, G. (Ed.). (1988). *Working with people*. London: Routledge.
Fransella, F. (1981). Nature babbling to herself: The self characterization as a therapeutic tool. In H. Bonarius, R. Holland, & S. Rosenberg (Eds.), *Personal construct psychology: Recent advances in theory and in practice.* New York: St. Martin's Press.
Leitner, L.M. (1985). Interview methodologies for construct elicitation: Searching for the core. In F. Epting & A.W. Landfield (Eds.), *Anticipating personal construct psychology.* Lincoln: University of Nebraska Press.
Thompson, M. (1989). *On art and therapy.* London: Virago Press.
White, M., & Epson, D. (1990). *Narrative means to therapeutic ends.* London: Pergamon.

Helping Clients to Retell Their Stories

Beck, A.T., Rush, A.J., Shaw, B.T., & Emery, G. (1979). *Cognitive therapy of depression.* New York: Guilford.
Berne, E. (1964). *Games people play.* London: Penguin.
Blows, M., & Srinivasan, S. (1991). *Studies in meditation.* Melbourne: Hill of Content Press.
Crose, R. (1990). Reviewing the past in the here and now: Using gestalt therapy techniques with life review. *Journal of Mental Health Counselling, 12,* 279–287.
Dalley, T., & Case, C. (1992). *The handbook of art therapy.* London: Routledge.
Ellis, A. (1979). Rational-emotive therapy and cognitive behaviour therapy: Similarities and differences. *Cognitive Therapy and Research, 4,* 325–340.
Epting, F.R., & Nazario, A. (1987). Designing a fixed role therapy: Issues, techniques and modifications. In R.A. Niemeyer & G.J. Niemeyer (Eds.), *A casebook in personal construct therapy.* New York: Springer.
Fagan, N.J., & Shepherd, I.L. (1971). *Gestalt therapy now.* New York: Harper & Row.
Freud, S. (1925). *The collected papers of Sigmund Freud.* London: Hogarth.
Gendlin, E.T. (1981). *Focussing.* New York: Bantam.
Gottschalk, L.A. (1985). *How to understand and analyse your own dreams.* Berkeley, CA: Art Reproduction Press.
Jennings, S. (1987). *Drama therapy.* London: Routledge.
Kelly, G.A. (1955). *The psychology of personal constructs.* New York: Norton.*
Kendall, P.C. (Ed.). (1985). *Advances in cognitive-behavioural research and therapy.* New York: Academic.
Mahrer, A.H. (1986). *Therapeutic experiencing.* New York: Norton.
Rubin, R.J. (Ed.). (1978). *Bibliotherapy sourcebook.* Phoenix: Onyx.
Rubin, J.A. (1987). *Approaches to art therapy.* New York: Brunner/Mazel.
Rudestam, K.E. (1980). *Methods of self change.* Monterey, CA: Brooks/Cole.

Viney, L.L. (1988). Psychotherapy as reconstruction. *International Journal of Personal Construct Psychology, 1,* 37–48.

Viney, L.L. (1989). *Images of illness,* Malabar, FL: Krieger.

Webster, J.D., & Cappeliez, P. (1993). Reminiscence and autobiographical memory: Complimentary contexts for cognitive aging research. *Developmental Review, 13,* 54–91.

Wolpe, J.P. (1969). *The practice of behaviour therapy.* Elmsford, NY: Pergamon.

Worden, W. (1991). *Grief counselling and grief therapy.* London: Routledge.

Yablonsky, L. (1981). *Psychodrama.* New York: Gardner.

Ending Therapy

Bannister, D. (1983). The internal politics of psychotherapy. In D. Pilgrim (Ed.), *Psychology and psychotherapy.* London: Routledge & Kegan Paul.*

Epting, F.R. (1984). *Personal construct counselling and psychotherapy.* New York: Wiley.

Landfield, A.W., & Epting, F.R. (1987). *Personal construct psychology: Clinical personality assessment.* New York: Human Sciences.

Pilgrim, D. (Ed.). (1983). *Psychology and psychotherapy.* London: Routledge & Kegan Paul.

EXERCISES

1. Identify the main psychological issues you deal with in beginning therapy with a client. Would it be helpful to deal with others? Which ones?
2. Use the three person comparison to identify both poles of some constructs of a client of yours.
3. Use writing a self-characterization to do the same.
4. Select a client of yours whose changes in action patterns appear to be blocked. Use the ABC Model to identify which of his or her construing is preventing change.
5. Select a client whose construing is loose and use analysis of his or her construing to tighten it.
6. Select a client whose construing is tight and use dream analysis, "empty chair," or art therapy to loosen it.
7. Show how you helped a client of yours to recognize him- or herself as a creator of his or her own constructs and therefore able to choose to change them.
8. Identify the main psychological issues you deal with in ending therapy with a client. Would it be helpful to deal with others? Which ones?

11

Some Therapeutic Strategies for Groups

I now want to consider some therapeutic strategies for working with groups of clients. This is because although personal construct psychology is sometimes accused of being very individually and personally oriented, to the exclusion of social and interpersonal aspects of clients, this is not so. Personal construct therapy is both concerned with the interpersonal functioning of clients and able to provide ways of working with clients in groups with a focus on these interpersonal processes. In this chapter, I look first at the constructivist ideas and strategies that are used for group work. These ideas start with the goals and functions of personal construct group work. Two different accounts of the cycles through which such group work may go as they develop are provided, followed by an account of the two personal construct theory assumptions that underlie this group work. The notion that good interpersonal functioning is crucial to the effective psychological functioning of clients is introduced, together with support for this notion from a number of recent writers about personal construct therapy. Some research studies that have shown personal construct group therapy to be effective with a wide range of clients will also be reviewed.

I then describe the strategies that are used in doing personal construct group work. These strategies include choices about the goals or purposes of this work and the decisions about group membership that need to be made along with the theoretical reasons for them. Structure is very important to personal construct groups and some alternative strategies that are used for developing group structure are considered. The leadership role taken in this group is also provided, as are some suggestions about how constructivist group work may best be reported.

These suggestions include the themes of group construction that emerge, the group processes that lead to them, and the emotional reactions. There are also tests of construing, which are started at first by the group leaders and later by the group members. These categories are then used to describe two examples of group therapy: young men who had been referred with a diagnosis of having HIV or AIDS and young people who were being encouraged to take fewer risks. The goals of the first group were to minimize the impact of ill health, whereas goals for the second group were to prevent illness and injury.

IDEAS AND STRATEGIES FOR PERSONAL CONSTRUCT GROUP WORK

Goals and functions of personal construct group work need to be discussed. Personal construct group therapy can be seen as providing even greater opportunities for testing construct systems for clients than does individual therapy. This is because of the greater range of feedback about how each member is perceived by other members and because of the controlled conditions in which these tests can be conducted. Personal construct group therapists find the therapeutic processes in group work identified by Yalom (1995) useful. The most important of these are hope, the sharing of information and emotions, and the expression of emotions or catharsis. Recognizing the similarities of the experiences of other group members to ones' own, altruism, imitative behavior, testing of vicarious solutions to problems, and the reliving of family problems in the group are also important. Personal construct group therapists have, however, their own descriptions of group therapeutic processes that merit mention here (Winter, 1992). These include opportunities for the group members to develop better discrimination, to examine their preemptive or stereotype-like constructs, and to add to their ability to understand the thoughts, emotions, and beliefs of a wider range of other people. A helpful dispersion of dependency, rather than relying on only a few people for help, can also be encouraged in group therapy. The general climate of a personal construct group provides validation for many of its members' constructs, with the uncritical acceptance and understanding of others being the context of construct system testing here as it is for individual therapy. Indeed, invalidation has been shown to be more effective when it comes from group members who have provided a climate of validation of the construing of others (Catina, Tschuschke, & Winter, 1989).

Personal construct groups, as they reconstrue, go through *cycles of sharing of construing and individuation of construing*. Some writers have even described these cycles as stages. However, as we saw in relation to bereavement (in Chapter 5), the psychological functioning that is occcurring is considered to be, in personal construct psychology, not so much in stages as in interweaving processes or cycles. One account of the cycles of such group work (Koch, 1985) describes them in this way: (a) searching for commonality and validation, (b) clarification of differences and reciprocal elaboration of construing, and (c) development of the relationships of individual members to the group, together with recognition of their individuality. Another account of these cycles (Llewelyn & Dunnett, 1987) presents them as follows: (a) cohesiveness and mutual support, (b) self-disclosure and attempts to construe each other's construing, (c) interactions that focus on particular constructs, (d) active experimentation within the group, and (e) setting homework for one another to try experimentation outside the group. Therapeutic experimentation in this group setting can, as in individual therapy, come from a wide range of other theories. They can include, for example, drawing, games, enactment of written scripts, role play with role reversal, reflecting on the group process using videos, considering their own and others' self-characterizations, and using the dyadic sharing of the interpersonal transactional group (Landfield & Rivers, 1975; R.A. Neimeyer, 1988). Group therapy processes, like the processes of individual personal construct therapy, are based on reconstruction.

Central to personal construct group process are two important *ideas about interpersonal relationships* from the theory underlying it. The first of these has been described as the sociality corollary (Kelly, 1955, p. 95). It states that "to the extent to which one person construes the construction processes of another, he [or she] may play a role in the social process involving another." This means that people can only interact effectively with others when they behave according to how they construe those others to construe and not according to their own constructions. This means that people come to understand others only when they come to see them as fellow construers. For young people who have difficulty doing this, enactment and role play can make it possible to do so. The other central idea is contained in the commonality corollary (Kelly, 1955, p. 90). It states that "to the extent that one person construes an event like another, their psychological processes will be similar." There will then be some commonality and sharing in the construing of people that helps to make communication between them possible. In group therapy, such shared construing is of course emphasized, as is the effects of others on the personal construing of any event (Dalton & Dunnett, 1993). From this approach, psychological well-being can be defined as the ability to experiment with shared construing, as well as with personal construing, together with the ability to take a perspective on events and not interpret them literally (Koch, 1985). Even emotions, such as guilt and shame, are now described as having social as well as personal origins (Mascolo, 1994). Group therapy is therefore especially useful to adolescents and to others who need to test and improve their interpersonal functioning because it provides opportunities to develop these capacities.

Shared construing and being able to take the perspective of another are important aspects of psychological well-being. There is, however, a developing body of work by Leitner and his colleagues (Faidley & Leitner, 1993; Leitner & Dill-Standiford, 1993) that suggests that people, in order to live rich and meaningful lives, need to able to relate to others not only distantly, but also intimately. Such close relationships require of clients, and therapists, interpersonal empathy, which is made up of a range of abilities. These abilities, which therapists encourage in their clients, include discrimination or the capacity to construe differences between other people and evaluate them in the light of their own construct systems (Leitner & Pfenninger, 1994). These abilities also include flexibility when interpersonal interactions do not proceed as planned, thereby developing alternative constructions about those interactions. Creativity is important here also because clients need to be able to create new ways of making sense of other people because those other people are constantly changing. Responsibility requires clients to be able to examine their own construct systems using the point of reference of the other person in the intimate relationship. Openness consists of willingness, when clients' constructs are invalidated by events, to reconstrue. Commitment to the other person in an intimate relationship also means agreeing to continue to validate his or her construing over time. Courage involves clients having a clear understanding of their own constructs about intimate relationships. When these relationships do not continue without problems, as they often do not, our clients need to be able to show forgiveness, requiring reconstruction of themselves and of the other person, in order to continue their relationships. Reverence is the final important capacity that has been identified. It involves awareness in clients that they are are being allowed, in an intimate relationship with another person, to validate their most central and influential and therefore most easily threatened constructs.

The outcomes of *evaluation studies for personal construct group work* are now reported. This group therapy has been shown to be effective with a wide range of clients using research designs including control groups with no group therapy (Winter, 1992). Some of the earliest work was with undifferentiated but hospitalized psychiatric patients who were found to change their construing of self after group work (Winter & Trippett, 1977). Stutterers were also early to experience the benefits of such group work in which they came to recognize the need for and to work on the development of construing of themselves as fluent people (Dalton, 1980). Depressives have also been found after group work to dilate their constricted construing (Winter, 1985). Women who were adult survivors of incestuous abuse have also been found to benefit from personal construct group work in terms of their construing of others and of their social adjustment (Harter, Alexander, & Neimeyer, 1988). Group therapy with people who are living with AIDS and voluntary AIDS caregivers (Viney, Allwood, & Stillson, 1991) has been shown to reduce the levels of their all too appropriate anxiety (Viney, Walker, & Crooks, 1995). Group work with acting-out adolescents helped them to become more aware of their self-construing and the role of others in validating this, as well as to lessen the confusion in their self-construing (Jackson, 1990).

DOING CONSTRUCTIVIST GROUP WORK

The main goal of constructivist group work is to enable group members to elaborate and extend their systems of construing. This elaboration can be carried out through validation or invalidation, loosening or tightening, dilation or constriction, or abstraction or concretization of some part of their construct systems. This can involve confirmation or disconfirmation and making their interpretations variable or more precise, broader or more specific, or more event based or generalizeable. Such group therapy should lead to the achievement of the same goals as in individual therapy. These goals include, of course, making the meanings of clients explicit, developing alternate stories within therapy, and changing their patterns of action. In group therapy, because of the greater opportunities available to the group members an even greater range of more viable choices, the last of the four goals, emerges for them than from individual therapy (Papanek, 1964).

A number of aspects of *group membership* now need to be considered. Personal construct groups can have from 6 to 20 members, with 6 to 12 members being the most common. Groups should be composed of a variety of clients with different experiences and views of the world. Although these groups start with sharing (Ryle & Lipshitz, 1976), they move on to differentiation of construing, which is aided by including such diversity (Alexander & Follette, 1985). Selection of individual group members should, it seems, be based on their ability to change their construing and to have an extensive enough construct system to begin to understand something of those of others (Winter, 1992). It also helps if the construing of the selected group members is not too tight, or precise, in terms of its interpretations and predictions. Other criteria for selection as group members has also been said to be the abilities to understand others and to form lasting intimate relationships. Because many clients are referred for group therapy precisely because they seem to lack these capacities, there may be no group work at all if we could work only with clients who already have these abilities. Selection of members on the basis of a lack of these qualities, but a demonstrated potential for them, seems useful. Potential abilities of this kind may have been demonstrated by our clients only rarely, with only a few other people and some time ago. Participation in these groups should be voluntary.

Structure is an integral part of personal construct group work because greater structure of such groups has been found to be linked with more therapeutic movement rather than less (G.J. Neimeyer & Merluzzi, 1991). Such groups are usually short, with perhaps 10 sessions, so that a group of 20 sessions would be considered long (Winter, 1992). The tasks that provide structure are selected in order to experiment with the current construing, or test the construct systems, of the group members. These tasks must extend the range of that construing a little so as to avoid anxiety, but do not require an inconveniently demanding leap of the members who will find this too difficult. The tasks are selected initially by the leader but, as the intimacy and spontaneity of the group develops, they can be selected jointly by leaders and group members. It is also helpful to involve all of the group members in reflecting on what has happened in the group sessions and on what experiments may be useful for the next session.

Such tasks may include the interpersonal transaction group (Landfield & Rivers, 1975). It involves five steps: (a) group members identify their moods, write them on labels, and share what is written on those labels with others; (b) they talk with only one other person in response to a question asked by the group leaders; (c) they move to another dyad and share those answers again with another individual; (d) they continue to share this response with all the other group members, one at a time; and (e) they identify their new moods, write them on labels, and share those labels again with the entire group. Questions that group leaders can choose to have answered can be: "Who am I?", "How can I give help to others and seek help from them?", "When do I feel safe and when do I not?", and "What would I most like to say to each group member?" Completing the five steps leads to increased understanding of one another's perspective and construing without requiring group members to take the center of the stage in order to disclose in front of the whole group. The interpersonal transaction group can be employed as a structuring task for all of the group sessions. Leaders can begin with the question: "Who am I?" in the first session. They can then turn to other questions related to the anxiety generated by events beyond the construct systems of the group members and, perhaps, to threats to their most central and influential constructs about relating to others.

Because group work is useful with adolescents, it is important to consider what structuring tasks may be helpful for them. Group members and their leaders could all be transported to Galaxy 21, a changing world where the familiar and unfamiliar live together. Many tests of construct systems can be made on such a galaxy. This task has been based on the "Magic Garden" for group work with younger children (Agnew, 1985). The Magic Garden, as it has been described, contains fairies who can do exciting and surprising things for the children who visit. Again, the combination of familiar and unfamiliar is central. Another structuring task for younger group members could involve role play of common but problematic interactions with others, such as negotiating a group decision or dealing with a point of conflict Such enactment and role reversal will aid in helping group members to better understand the construing of others, as well as their own. These tasks can also provide helpful structures for personal construct group work with adult and elderly clients.

The *role of the group leaders* also needs to be discussed. The group leaders, as well as choosing the structure of the group, ensure that there is a general climate of validation of construing within the group. They also fulfill a number of other functions. These functions include understanding the constructs of the group members and showing that they do so, as well as providing feedback to them which confirms and supports the construing of the group. These leaders are also involved in accepting and being interested in (or validating) the group members (Koch, 1985). They have the goals of making meanings more explicit, developing alternate stories, changing action patterns, and widening the ranges of choices for their group members to keep in mind. They work to make the construing of their group members broader and more abstract. This process helps the members to integrate their learnings into as abstract a level of their construct systems as possible in order to ensure future access to them when as wide a range of concrete events as possible is encountered. The role of the leader is thus a very important and complex one. Two group leaders are therefore recommended, especially if the group is large. Research has indicated that it is the group members who see the group leader as more similar to their parents who show more movement than those who see them as less similar (Koch, 1983). Transference, of early stories about old events to these new events, is therefore helpful in this personal construct group therapy as it is in individual personal construct therapy.

A standard form for *reporting the progress of each group session* is useful. These reports can include (a) the goals and functions of the group work, (b) the members, (c) the leaders, (d) the themes that have emerged, (e) the group process that produced those themes, (f) the emotions experienced by the participants, and (g) the experiments started by the leaders and by the group members. The goals of the group can be considered in terms of the testing, and therefore the elaboration of the constructs systems of the group members, and the specific functions that a particular group may be formed in order to achieve. In the two examples of group work that I describe, their functions were different. One was concerned with treatment and the other with prevention. Information needs to be provided about both the clients who make up the group and the leader or leaders. The themes that are considered are themes of construction. They indicate the focus of the group as they seek to make their own experiences meaningful. The group processes give rise to these themes. Although group themes can be found as noun-based descriptions of what has transpired, process focuses more on action and so is verb based. It is through these group processes that reconstruction can be seen to occur. It involves both the sharing of group members and individuation. It is also useful to record the tests or experiments that are carried out by both the group: leaders and the group members. I now use this form of reporting to describe two applications of this form of group therapy with which I have been involved.

PERSONAL CONSTRUCT GROUP WORK WITH MEN WHO ARE LIVING WITH AIDS: AN EXAMPLE

This group work was developed in order to meet some of the needs of men who have been diagnosed with HIV or have developed AIDS-related illnesses (Viney et al., 1991). These men experienced much distress, including anxiety, anger, and helplessness, because so much of their past construing was being invalidated by the events of diagnosis and illness.

The main *goal* of this group work was to help these men to reconstrue these troubling, and in some cases devastating, events in their lives. Those of us who use this constructivist perspective see much of the distress of these men as arriving from their problems in making their new lives meaningful to themselves and in anticipating effectively what was going to happen to them. Invalidation of their old ways of construing was rife from lovers, families, friends, and health professionals. It was for this reason, then, that reconstruction was needed by them. They also needed to recognize their own ability to construe and reconstrue. Because invalidation was also intrusive and common for them, increasing their sources of validation for their new construing was also seen as important. This could first be achieved within the group through improvements in their interpersonal functioning and in their learning to use a wider range of source of validations. It was also planned to achieve this goal, after the group had ended, by carrying their new social awareness and capacities over into the lives of the members.

The *members* who participated were from a gay community much affected by HIV. Many of these men were young and well-educated professionals, all of whom admitted they were gay to their friends and families. Their participation was voluntary. The group consisted of eight men who met for ten 1½-hr sessions with one group leader.

The *leader* was a young, gay social worker named John who was also diagnosed with HIV. He consulted weekly with me about his group leadership. The first concern that he shared with me during supervision involved the care with which he needed to make this offer of group therapy to the prospective members. Several of the men whom we saw as being both able to benefit and willing to take the risks involved in such experimentation refused. We were able, after considerable discussion both with these men and between ourselves, to realize that they were seeing our offer as invalidation of their central constructs about being competent and able to look after their own psychological welfare. We noticed, too, that this seemed particularly to be the case for men who had recently gone through the very difficult process of acknowledging their sexual preference and establishing a gay identity. We then learned to make our offer so as to complement and confirm the sense of competence that they had developed through this process rather than undermining it. Confidentiality was another important issue for these men, of which John and I remained well aware.

The major *themes of construction* that emerged from the group process with these men were those of awareness, self-construing, emotions, and relationships. The group members were surprised by their own lack of awareness of many aspects of their own lives. Time was one of these, with the members concerned about how they had been taking it for granted until now, and how perception of time can vary with people and occasions. Their continued attempts to construe themselves centred on "How do I really feel about myself?" and "What does being a man mean?" Their reconstruing of their relationships focused on communication problems as well as on the need to take responsibility in intimate relationships and yet also assert their own rights. They began to become aware, as well, of some of the repeated patterns of their construing. They saw some of their current close relationships as being like those they had had with their own parents and how they were repeating those relationships in other situations. They also focused on the theme of trusting others not only initially, but also throughout the group sessions. The members found it helpful to reflect on these themes themselves at the end of each session.

The *group processes* were as follows. One of the many types of construing shared by the group members were the group rules that were tried and tested as the group began. Three rules were accepted and acted on by this group: (a) maintaining confidentiality, (b) being honest, and (c) working in the here and now. They were also aware of sharing construing about gay pride. However, as the group sessions continued, greater differentiation of the group members started to emerge. This became particularly apparent as they dealt with issues of identity, illness, and health. They found, for example in the area of illness, that they had had very different meaning for illness and how it should be handled by others. Because much of this construing originally came from the construing of their family of origin, those individualizing or differentiating aspects of their lives also came to be recognized as representing the very different early experiences that they had had.

The first *emotions* that were expressed by these group members were positive, with acknowledgment of acceptance and openness. Evidence of some validation of their construing was then available. As the group sessions continued, however, it was their fear of the negative emotions arising from invalidation that became apparent. In the early sessions, such emotional reactions were avoided. As the sessions progressed, though, the negative emotion of guilt began to dominate discussions. This guilt was often linked with their acting with a partner in a close relationship in ways that were in conflict with some of their most central constructs about how they should behave with others. Some anger also began to show but at first it was directed at distant targets, like governments and AIDS organizations, rather than at the AIDS-related illnesses that were threatening them. In the later sessions, however, there was more expression of anger at this target.

The *group experiments* conducted by the leader helped the group members to focus on the content of their constructs and on the implications of those constructs for how they behaved. Answering questions about expectations of the group was one way of securing construct content, whereas the simple three-person comparison that was the basis of the Repertory Grid Techniques was another. Laddering and pyramiding, asking the questions "Why is this important to you?" and "How did this effect things?", were used to provide more information about their underlying construct systems and their use. The implications of the content of their construing were largely explored through enactment. Enactment involved acting out events in order to come to reinterpret them. This occurred partly through the acting of specific dialogues of conflict between men, written by the group leader for that purpose. Another involved fixed-role therapy. The experiments that were created by the group members were of a different kind and later in the sessions. They differed in form from person to person depending on experiments that were needed to extend the construct system of each member. One member experimented with allowing himself to feel angry and another with how close he permitted himself to become to another group member.

Several *outcomes* of the group work became apparent. At the end of the 10 group sessions, the members showed considerable evidence of reconstruction. They were beginning to find new ways of making sense of and valuing their new, post-AIDS lives. They were also beginning to see themselves as less dependent on life events but as creators of their own construing. They were also beginning to see themselves as recreators of their own construing. During group sessions, the group members received considerable validation from other group members and from the group leader for their new construing. They had learned about the value of that validation from others and began to increase their ability to seek for it and accept it. They emerged from the group with a better understanding of the importance of access to a range of social supports in their lives.

The *reflections of the group leader* need to be reported. During supervision with me, John and I identified four types of difficulty in the group process. One had to do with the problems that some of the group members had in becoming aware of their own feelings. Another had to do with the fear of self-exposure that some experienced, which tended to interfere with their group participation. Some feared to admit that they construed themselves as weak, whereas others feared rejection from others. We were also concerned about the impact of the many political issues surrounding AIDS relating to discrimination, drug trials, and prevention, such that it was sometimes difficult for John to contain the communications to within the group because there was so much going on outside the group that was both engaging and frustrating.

We were also able to identify some aspects of John's construing that needed monitoring during group sessions. We had believed before the group that because John was male, gay, and HIV it would empower him as leader for this kind of group. These similarities did seem to make it easier for him to get the group processes started and to secure trust from the group members. However, John did find, as the sessions continued, that he tended at times to identify with certain group members who were like him, and so ran the risk of not experimenting with them as effectively as he could. We also began to realize how important it was for him to be aware, before the group started, of his own construing of issues that were bound to be considered in the group, such as close relationships, identity, gay identity, illness, AIDS, and death. When he found that the group discussions of several of these issues did arouse some anxiety for him, we spent time together in supervision exploring his construing in those areas and the sources of validation he was using to support it.

GROUP WORK WITH RISK-TAKING ADOLESCENTS: ANOTHER EXAMPLE

This second example of personal construct group work was conducted with high-school adolescents with the goal of maintaining their health, especially in terms of sexually transmitted diseases (Viney, Truneckova, Weekes, & Oades, 1994). This work was carried out with adolescents in both schools and juvenile detention centers, but it is a school-based group that is reported here.

The main *goal* of this group work was to help the group members elaborate their construing of themselves and others, giving them more choices in how they related to others. However, in the context in which this group was run, better negotiation of current and future sexual relationships was especially intended. As well as this intention, the purpose was to preserve the health of these young people by helping them to negotiate better sexual encounters safe from sexually transmitted diseases.

The *members* consisted of 5 girls and 5 boys, all 15 or 16 years old. Although they came from the same school, they did not know one another before the group. Their participation was voluntary. The group met in a school room but not one usually used for classes. They met with two group leaders for 10 sessions.

The group *leaders* for this group were a young man, George, and a young woman, Nan, who were both school counselors. This meant that they had trained and worked as teachers before doing special courses in assessing and conducting individual counselling with school-age children.

Several major *themes of construction* emerged. The focus of the construing of these adolescent group members in the early group sessions were on testing the water, trust, and ownership of feelings. In the middle sessions, as they enacted some of the negotiations around sexual encounters, their themes dealt more with frustration, social gaffs, communication, and acceptance. In sessions later still, the focus was more on courage, growth, achievement, vulnerability, and strength. The group members joined with the leaders after the sessions in identifying some of these themes just as they were able to identify some of the group processes and emotions that had been expressed.

The *group processes* were as follows. Sharing processes, in which how much the group members seemed to have in common, were the initial group processes apparent for this group as they were for the older group. Also, this group expressed much of its commonality in terms of the rules that became explicit for conduct in the group. These rules were confidentiality, honesty, and trying to be open to one another's point of view. The individuating processes that were more apparent later in this group were particularly evident in the picture they chose to represent themselves when invited to do so by the group leaders. These images were a tree, a journey, a juggler, a clown, a fat man, a carpet, balloons, poppies, a butterfly, and a lion. Such choices made clear to them something of the different ways in which they were construing themselves.

The first *emotions* expressed by this group were also positive. They were togetherness and warmth. This meant that there was an early climate of validation or confirmation of construing in the group. There was also, however, evidence in the form of feelings of anxiety, fear, and frustration of some invalidation or disconfirmation. As the group sessions continued, there was still confusion, doubt, and shame and as the last sessions approached, even sadness. However, there was also hope, confidence, excitement, enjoyment, and much shared laughter.

Some of the *experiments* conducted by the two group leaders consisted of using pictures to represent the self, as I have described, and enactment of interactions between young people. These included acting out sexual negotiations with role reversal being helpful in beginning to understand the construing of the opposite-gender role. They also involved bringing a present to the group on its final session to represent what the group had meant to its members. The group members' experiments were of a different order, extending their construct systems by giving negative as well as positive feedback to other group members and trying out their own construing of the internal world of another.

Some useful *outcomes* of the group work can now be reported. The reconstruing that these younger group members achieved through group processes involved them in developing a greater understanding of their own construing, so adding to their awareness of self. They also came to understand the construing of the other members of the group more effectively, especially that of members of the opposite gender. They also began to see others as construers like themselves with similar thoughts and feelings, doubts, and fears. With this gain came greater confidence about the negotiation of relationships, both casual and intimate, including safer sexual ones.

The *reflections of the group leaders* are of interest. These group leaders, George and Nan, also worked with supervision from me. We used that supervision to ensure that they were continuing to use personal construct ideas as they conducted and reflected on the groups. We also monitored the understanding of group themes, processes, and emotions that were reported from the groups and carefully considered the experiments conducted and their outcomes. The leaders were concerned about the psychosocial maturity of some members of the group. They were also concerned at times that some members would not take the risks of self-exposure before the group sessions ended. Ten sessions of group process did prove long enough for them all to do so. We were also all concerned at times about whether a number of members would be able to develop any capacity to take on the perspective of another but in the time available they all did so.

In our supervisory discussions, we spent time on the rather different issues from the tendency to identify too easily with the group members that the first leader, John, experienced. With this group, there was more of a concern that the leaders were experiencing great differences from the group members in terms of maturity and culture. Some of the "in" language of the young group members, especially expressing emotions, was not known to us and we found that we needed to consult other young people of their age in order to fully understand some of their meanings.

DOING PERSONAL CONSTRUCT THERAPY WITH GROUPS OF CLIENTS

In this chapter, I have taken the ideas of personal construct therapy and applied them to working with groups of clients. The goals and functions of such groups and the stages or cycles of group processes that have been provided by fellow personal construct therapists have been examined and the major constructivist assumptions underlying group work. The reader has been alerted to some of the therapists who see group work as very important because psychological well-being can be defined in terms of capacities to perform social tasks. The research studies showing personal construct group therapy to be effective have also been reviewed. I have shown how personal construct group therapy can be conducted, in terms of its goals, and the membership and structure of groups. The role of the group leader and how personal construct group work can be reported have also been dealt with. So have two examples of group therapy for which supervision, using this form of report, has been provided.

In this section of this book, I have focused on strategies by which therapeutic reconstruction can be achieved. Chapter 10 was concerned, as in earlier chapters, with individual therapy. This chapter has been concerned with group therapy. It now remains for me to provide the last chapter of this book which, fittingly for one based on constructive theory, deals with the need for careful reflection by therapists on the processes of psychotherapy.

READINGS

Ideas and Strategies of Personal Construct Group Work

Catina, A., Tschuschke, V., & Winter, D. (1989). Self-reconstruction as a result of interaction in analytic group therapy. *Group Analysis, 22,* 59–62.

Dalton, P. (Ed.). (1980). *Approaches to the treatment of stuttering.* London: Croom Helm.

Dalton, P., & Dunnett, G. (1993). *Living with personal construct psychology.* Chichester: Wiley.

Faidley, A.J., & Leitner, L.M. (1993). *Assessing experience in psychotherapy: Personal construct alternatives,* Westport, CT: Praeger.

Harter, S., Alexander, P.C., & Neimeyer, P.C. (1988). Long term effects of incestuous child abuse in college women: Social adjustment, social cognition and family characteristics. *Journal of Consulting & Clinical Psychology, 56,* 5–8.

Jackson, S. (1990). A personal construct therapy group for adolescents. In P. Maitland (Ed.), *Personal construct theory, deviancy and social work.* London: Centre for Personal Construct Psychology.

Kelly, G.A. (1955). *The psychology of personal constructs.* New York: Norton.

* Most useful readings.

Koch, H. (1985). Group psychotherapy. In E. Button (Ed.), *Personal construct theory and mental health*. Beckenham: Croom Helm.*

Landfield, A.W., & Rivers, P.C. (1975). An introduction to interpersonal transaction and rotating dyads. *Psychotherapy, 12,* 366–374.

Leitner, L.M., & Dill-Standiford, T. (1993). Resistance in experiential personal construct psychotherapy: Theoretical and technical struggles. In L.M. Leitner & G. Dunnet (Eds.), *Critical issues in personal construct psychology*. Malabar, FL: Krieger.

Leitner, L.M., & Pfenninger, D.T. (1994). Sociality and optimal functioning. *Journal of Constructivist Psychology, 7,* 119–136.*

Llewelyn, S., & Dunnett, G. (1987). The use of personal construct theory in groups. In R.A. Neimeyer & G.J. Neimeyer (Eds), *Personal construct theory casebook*. New York: Springer.

Mascolo, M. (1994). Towards a social constructivist psychology: The case of self-evaluative emotional development. *Journal of Constructivist Psychology, 7,* 107–119.

Neimeyer, R.A. (1988). Clinical guide-lines for conducting interpersonal transaction groups. *International Journal of Personal Construct Psychology, 1,* 181–190.*

Viney, L.L., Allwood, K., & Stillson, L. (1991). Reconstructive group therapy for HIV seropositive patients. *Counselling Psychology Quarterly, 4,* 243–254.

Viney, L.L., Walker, B., & Crooks, L. (1995). Anxiety in community-based AIDS care givers before and after counselling. *Journal of Clinical Psychology, 51,* 274–279.

Winter, D. (1985). Group therapy with depressives: A personal construct theory perspective. *International Journal of Mental Health, 13,* 3–5, 67–85.

Winter, D. (1992). *Personal construct psychology in clinical practice*. London: Routledge.*

Winter, D.A., & Trippett, C.J. (1977). Serial change in group psychotherapy. *British Journal of Medical Psychology, 50,* 341–348.

Yalom, I. (1995). *The theory and practice of group psychotherapy.* New York: Basic Books.

Doing Constructivist Group Work

Agnew, J. (1985). Childhood disorders or the ventures of children. In E. Button (Ed.), *Personal construct theory and mental health*. London: Croom Helm.*

Alexander, S., & Follette, V. (1985). Personal constructs in group treatment of incest. In R.A. Neimeyer & G.J. Neimeyer (Eds.), *Personal construct therapy casebook*. New York: Springer.

Koch, H.C.H. (1983). Changes in personal construing in the psychotherapy group and a control group. *British Journal of Medical Psychology, 56,* 245–255.

Neimeyer, G.J., & Merluzzi, T.V. (1991). Group structure and group process:

Explorations in therapeutic sociality. *Small Group Behaviour, 13,* 150–164.

Papanek, H. (1964). Bridging dichotomies through group psychotherapy. *Journal of Individual Psychology, 20,* 38–47.

Ryle, A., & Lipshitz, S. (1976). An intensive case study of a therapeutic group. *British Journal of Psychiatry, 128,* 581–587.

Personal Construct Group Work With Examples

Viney, L.L., Truneckova, D., Weekes, P., & Oades, L. (1994). *Personal construct group therapy for adolescents.* Paper presented at the Australian Psychological Society Conference, Wollongong.

EXERCISES

1. People have described personal construct therapy as being based on personal rather than interpersonal ideas. Debate whether this is so or not.
2. If you have conducted group therapy using other therapeutic approaches, does this constructivist account of group work aid you in understanding what occurred?
3. Select some of the structures for personal construct groups that can help you and your clients achieve your goals.
4. When you conduct some personal construct group therapy, does it show the cycles of commonality and individuality that have been described?
5. When you conduct such group therapy, what themes of construction emerge? What group processes? What emotions? What experiments?

VI

REFLECTIONS

12

Being an Effective Personal Construct Therapist

This account of personal construct therapy began with a description of its unique ideas and strategies and a comparison of this therapy with other therapies (Chapter 1). I then considered constructivist ideas about people, for example, the central role of subjectivity, the importance of meaning (especially created meanings), and the human abilities to act as if (Chapter 2). This account of personal construct therapy continued with the major constructivist ideas about therapy (Chapter 3). The view that both therapists (Chapter 4) and clients (Chapter 5) are construers has also been made clear. This is also true of the notion that we can all reconstrue, especially when this involves retelling the stories which we tell each other in therapy.

The aspects of personal construct therapy that I have identified so far have to do with the way therapists make sense of clients and themselves; that is, they are conceptual. As was indicated at the beginning of this book, these ideas are central to personal construct therapy. There are other aspects of this therapy, however, that are more practical and they too are represented in this account of it. They include some of the goals of that therapy (Chapter 7), the importance of the retelling of stories (Chapter 8), and the shared roles of clients and therapists working together to achieve these goals (Chapter 9). They also include some answers to the question about what to do in therapy with individual clients (Chapter 10), including both how to understand the construing of clients and how to help them to understand and retell their stories. Also provided is an account of some of what I do in therapy with groups of clients (Chapter 11).

I now want to finish this book on personal construct therapy by examining how therapists can work toward becoming more effective therapists using the ideas of this approach. This can best be achieved by again applying these ideas to our own conduct as therapists. Monitoring our own construing then becomes the first step in this process. This self-monitoring can include the content of our construing and its process, together with using whatever strategies we can to maximize awareness of these aspects of our construing. We also need to monitor the ethical positions we take in relation to our clients. This can include the values that inform our models of moral reasoning, the variety of such values that clients and even other therapists can have, the balance of powers in the therapeutic relationship, and our stances on some ethical issues central to therapy. Monitoring our own contribution to therapy is also important. I deal with the influence of my life experiences and how I create my own ways of functioning as a therapist, as well as the importance of my providing for my clients clear feedback and credible and useful stories. We also need to come to consider carefully our own goals and strategies. Acknowledging that we learn from our clients is also important because our construing is constantly changing. Supervision is also important here. In my discussion of many of these ways to become a more effective therapist, I use examples from therapy with the clients that I have described in some detail in earlier chapters of this book.

SELF-MONITORING THE CONSTRUING OF THE THERAPIST

The Construing Content

The *content of my construing* and that of other personal construct therapists, needs to be monitored. Because personal construct therapists use a reflexive theory, all of our strategies for making ourselves more effective therapists must be based on the ideas that we use to make sense of our clients. In Chapter 4, I showed that this is both necessary and possible. Monitoring our own construing is the first step in that process and a focus on the content of that construing is the first of a number of different approaches to this task. There are also a number of ways in which this can be achieved. One involves comparing the content of the constructs that both we and our clients use to make some common aspects of our lives meaningful. When I was working with Christine, that anxious and depressed young married woman, her construing of her father was crucial to some aspects of that therapy. I considered carefully the similarities and differences in our construct content dealing with our fathers, using the similarities to help me to understand Christine' thoughts, feelings, and actions but keeping her differences from me clear in my mind so as not to impose my own construing on hers. Another way to consider the content of my construing is to examine the constructs that I am using to make sense of clients on the basis of the similarities I see between them and other earlier clients. With Frank, the middle-aged diabetic who had been referred for therapy by the courts for property damage, I at first interacted with him on the basis of the constructs I had built up about earlier clients who had been court referrals. As we met over a number of sessions, it became apparent that Frank's experiences and so his construing were unique and that I needed to listen very carefully to the stories he shared with me. Starting work with clients probably often involves us as therapists in functioning in this somewhat stereotypic fashion to begin with but moving on to understand the client in his or her individuality as quickly as possible.

There are three other aspects of the content of our construing that we also need to monitor. The first of these is using some of our construing of intimate relationships in our own lives to help our clients in understanding theirs. Christine, as a fairly recently married young woman, was still negotiating a balance in her relationship with her husband of being there and not being there for one another. She was experiencing some of her first occasions when the needs of both herself and her husband for support and validation were very great simultaneously. When asked by her about my own experiences of this difficult situation, I was able to give a reply based on some optimism about the need to acknowledge and deal with these occasions. This optimism was based on their being only a small part, so far anyway, of my own most intimate relationship. Countertransference is another crucial aspect of therapist self-monitoring. This involves the transfer of stories from the therapists' early experiences with people to events in the therapeutic relationship. It is possible for us to take into therapy some of our own problematic construing so that the therapy becomes about us rather than about our clients. Having been in therapy myself helps me to recognize when this occurs and such therapy is very strongly recommended for personal construct therapists (Kelly, 1955; Kenny, 1988). Knowing that I can quite easily slip into depression and guilt with a depressed client, for example, means that I am careful about how many depressed clients I see and to schedule them early in the week when I am stronger. Apart from this ability to recognize parallel reconstruing like this in myself and my client, therapy for would-be therapists can provide us with a clearer sense of the intimate relationship of therapy. Such therapy also provides opportunities for self-understanding and personal growth. The third aspect of the content of our construing is experiences with clients that are beyond the range of our construct system given its content. I know that this is occurring when I feel uneasy or anxious during therapy. Elderly Ethel, who was herself initially anxious and withdrawn, gave me some uneasy moments of this kind. On reflection, this proved to be because the content of her integrity-based construing, which was age appropriate for her, was unfamiliar to me as a younger person.

The Construing Processes

The *processes of our construing* involve the ways in which we use our constructs rather than their content. We need, as therapists, to make our own construct system as permeable as possible (Epting, 1984). That is, when I work as a therapist I like to be using constructs that can quickly make sense of events that are new to us. Just as it is apparent that the construct systems of both clients and therapists need to be permeable, there is another aspect of constructivist experience that is ideally shared by both therapists and clients. Therapists, too, need to be able to function as if. That is, helpful to us and of course also to our clients if we are not easily trapped into a naïve realist view of the world in which our experiences and opportunities are given rather than constructed. There are always alternate views available of any event. It is also important that we develop a construct system that is subsuming that can make sense of the construct systems of our clients (Kelly, 1955). We need such a system that enables us to make sense of the construct systems of our clients rather than setting up a different system of constructs in competition with theirs. I have described how that process of subsuming Christine's constructs with mine worked with her.

We also need to recognize when our construing is confused in therapy. Although this can result from my own inability to understand my clients, it can sometimes be a confusion that reflects the inability of my clients themselves to interpret and anticipate events effectively. This proved to be the case with Frank, with whom I did begin to feel confused. This confusion actually turned out to reflect the lack of meaning and inability to predict of Frank's world, his internal chaos. It is also important for me as a therapist to remember that some of my own construing may be preverbal (Kenny, 1987). This became apparent to me when I worked with a client, who has not been mentioned before. She was recently divorced and our first agreed goal for therapy was to prepare her for more successful intimate relationships in the future. In response to my request to keep records of her dream to be shared with me, she produced one that I saw as bearing on our goal and on the relationship that we were trying to develop in therapy. Her account of this dream was, briefly, as follows:

> I was walking into a bar, and there were figures like people sitting on bar stools turned away from me. As I moved towards them, they turned towards me. And the hands they reached out were skeleton hands with shrivelled and rotting skin on them, and their faces were just skeletons.

She showed no emotion as she told me this. My reaction to the extreme desolation of this image was close to panic. I completed our session as best I could and reflected with the help of an experienced therapist colleague on how it must have touched preverbal construing of rejection and death of mine, leading to the intense emotional reaction I experienced. On the basis of that dream, this client and I revised our goal to focus more on her development of a personally satisfying lifestyle.

Awareness of Our Own Construing

Given the wide range of construing and stories about clients that we as therapists hold and the helpfulness of some and the unhelpfulness of others, it is clearly important for us to try to be *as aware of these constructs and stories as possible.* Supervision by other experienced therapists whom we can trust is invaluable in this process. I can check with those with whom I work in supervision the content of my own constructs, as I found I needed to do with Christine. I also need to check to see what culturally shared blind spots I may have, as I found in working with Frank. In this context of culturally shared blind spots, there is a marked lack of awareness of the constructs some therapists use to make sense of some kinds of clients. Elderly clients, like Ethel, provide an unfortunate example (Viney, 1993). In fact, relatively few training programs in clinical and counseling psychology, for example, even mention the elderly, let alone require supervised practical experience of therapy with them (Cohen & Cooley, 1983). Avoidance of elderly clients by mental health professionals is common, both in training and later in practice (Gatz & Pearson, 1988). Two emotional reactions of potential therapists to the elderly seems to be most likely to be responsible for this. One is that the elderly can present a severe threat to the core constructs of younger, healthy, cognitively alert therapists whom they remind that they, too, may be older, ill, and even cognitively impaired one day. The second emotional reaction of therapists that seems likely to lead to their avoidance of elderly clients may be guilt. In this reaction, again recognizing that they are younger, healthier, and more cognitively alert, they feel guilt because elderly clients do not share some of these enviable attributes. The most central and influential constructs of these potential therapists about how they relate to others require of them that they share their good fortune with others, and these attributes they cannot share.

Given the culture in which Western therapists work, there are many stereotypes and myths about the elderly that they can deceive themselves with so that therapy for elderly clients becomes to them neither necessary nor appropriate. These myths and stereotypes are often linked with descriptions of the elderly that degrade them, for example, "old man" or "little old lady." Such deceptions enable potential therapists for the elderly to see them as senile, generally incompetent, having lost their sexual potency, alienated, ill, and lacking control and flexibility (Rabbitt & Abson, 1991). If this is natural state of the elderly, psychotherapy cannot be helpful to them. Potential therapists who believe to accept these myths are therefore spared coming to terms with their own anxieties and guilt.

SELF-MONITORING OF THE ETHICAL POSITION OF THE THERAPIST

The Model of Moral Reasoning and Differences in Ethical Values

Three main principles are often cited as important for psychotherapists and as making up a *model of moral reasoning*. These principles are giving to and caring for clients, being just to clients, and respecting their autonomy (Beauchamp & Childless, 1983). Although these principles may meet some of the criteria for a model of moral reasoning, of being true for all and being consistent, for example (Steiner, Newall, & Garcia, 1984), there is not necessarily agreement about these principles. Although I accept these principles generally, I do not necessarily subscribe to them for all of my clients and on all occasions. Circumstances and construct systems can make them of different importance, it seems to me. I may also have some difficulty, even though I do see my first responsibility as to my clients, in them weighing up my responsibilities if they at times conflict with these responsibilities. Responsibilities to clients' families, to their referral sources and to government laws which require disclosure of some information revealed by clients, can also make for some difficult decision making for me.

It has been suggested that men and women may *differ in the ethical values* by which they live (Gilligan, 1982). Women tend to stress obligations to relationships with others that involve minimal pain for others and self, whereas men tend to stress people's rights to privacy and separateness from others. In the mature adult, both principles are ideally used together and perhaps that is what has occurred in the model of moral reasoning that I have just described. However, relatedness and separateness are two ethical principles that could easily be in conflict. As a woman therapist, I acknowledge the relatedness that has been at the center of my own model of moral reasoning for as long as I can remember, although more recently I have learned to acknowledge the human need for separateness too. I also must try to remain aware of the values of the different clients, communities, and cultures with which I work as I try to follow an ethical path. Religious beliefs can be linked to special beliefs about self, other people, and God and can influence the ethical courses that therapists choose to follow (Lawless, 1989). Therapists need to consider carefully how these ideas may influence our work with clients. We also need to acknowledge that we cannot avoid transmitting some of our ethical values to our clients during therapy sessions (Lakin, 1991). It is therefore essential that these values are both based on moral principles and useful for decision making in daily life.

The Balance of Power in Therapy

Personal construct therapists have, as I have shown, been concerned for some time about the *balance of power* in the therapeutic relationship. Although therapists who use other sets of ideas have tended to see themselves as the only experts in the health care interaction, personal construct therapists have acknowledged the special expertise of clients (Bannister, 1983). This has led to more empowering of clients when they deal with us in therapy. Our clients are in a better position to understand themselves, when compared with us, their therapists. There is hopefully a growing recognition that the autonomy of clients may be the most important value to influence and shape our interactions with them. It is, after all, clients who best understand their own constructs, goals, and values. The powerless "sick role" is inappropriate for clients and has unwanted emotional consequences for them. Clients learn to be, too, their own therapists, maintaining their own psychological well-being. There is a growing tendency in health care more generally for clients to be empowered to make decisions about and monitor their own treatment, even when that treatment is physical treatment for physical illness (World Health Organization, 1981). How much more appropriate and needed is this empowerment of our psychotherapy clients (Lakin, 1991). Such empowerment also needs to allow clients to refuse treatment, including psychotherapy (Mental Health Task Force, 1991).

Some Ethical Issues for Therapists

There are many ethical issues that must be of concern to us as therapists. *Informed consent* is an ethical standard required of all interventions by health care professionals (Fairbairn & Fairbairn, 1987), yet in psychotherapy it is not always possible to properly inform potential clients about what will happen in the course of their therapy. This is partly because, in personal construct therapy, given that both my clients and myself are constantly changing, anticipating exactly what will happen with us is difficult. It is also because, in the interaction between us before therapy, we are only beginning to establish our common construing and language that will take the full length of the therapy to develop. Effective communication by me before therapy of what is going to happen is difficult. One aspect of therapy I do try to make clear to all my clients before therapy is that they are likely to feel anxiety during it. Such anxiety occurs, of course, when clients begin to be aware of aspects of their experiences that are not made meaningful by their construct systems.

Another ethical issue of which I am constantly aware is *protecting the welfare of clients*. Studies of psychotherapists have shown that one regrettably common attack on their welfare is through sexual intimacy between therapist and client (Pope, 1990). For personal construct therapists to whom reconstruction within the therapeutic relationship is central to therapy, sexual intimacy during or after therapy is seen as serving only to validate the construing of the therapist and not helpful to the reconstruing of clients. Furthermore, it can prevent our clients' learning to use wider sources of validation of their construing that we are working with them to gain.

I also try to guarantee *confidentiality* of any information given by my clients to me in therapy. This promise helps to build trust and intimacy between us and also serves to protect the welfare of my clients. There are, however, some qualifications that I judge that I need ethically make to this guarantee. The first involves telling my clients, from the beginning of therapy, that I plan to share what happens between us with one or a small group of expert therapists with whom I need to reflect from time to time on what happens. To not do so would, I believe, be unethical. I also reserve the right to share certain kinds of information involving harm (e.g., through violence) to my client or other people with other professionals whose role it is to prevent this harm. So, although my ethical standards require that my client is my first concern, I am also mindful of my responsibilities to others. I do not make such disclosures, however, without discussing this fully with my client first. AIDS is facing therapists with some grave dilemmas of confidentiality (Ross, 1989). When clients have HIV, they can easily infect a sexual partner who has not tested positive. Some therapists have recommended breaching confidentiality to inform regular partners at least (Gray & Harding, 1988). Others believe that it is more ethical to work with the clients themselves to share their HIV status with their partners (Kain, 1988). These competing responsibilities are very difficult to resolve.

There are also ethical issues that we as therapists must be aware of because of the *different cultures in which we and our clients may live.* Sometimes these cultures are nationally and ethnically based (Dardenne & Mahtani, 1989; Sue, 1981) but others are based on gender and age (Lakin, 1991). In personal construct terms, cultures can be seen as sharing sets of constructs that are not shared by other cultures (Kalekin-Fischmann & Walker, 1995). Although sharing cultures with our clients can make it easier for us to start to work with them, it is possible for us to work with clients of other cultures. What we require of ourselves in this situation is to recognize the cultural differences in our construing and to try to understand and work within the culture in which our clients live.

SELF-MONITORING THE CONTRIBUTIONS TO THERAPY OF THE THERAPIST

Therapy Theory, Role, and Clarity

We choose both *the ideas* with which we work and *the therapist* role that we play. These are two contributions to all of our therapy for which we are responsible. The choices we make are also likely to be influenced by some of our own life experiences. My preference for the constructivist approach fits with the preferences I had even as a high-school history student. I found history taught as fact as somewhat dull but history taught as perceptions of what people may have experienced, supported with as much evidence as possible, much more exciting. It is from my mother that I not only learned this acknowledgment of the separateness of others from us, but also the capacity to bridge the gap between us through empathy. I also learned from her to value the as if worlds, so prized by personal construct therapists. It is from her, too, and probably much earlier in my life than I can remember, that I learned to experience the form of intimacy that I am now able to offer to those of my clients who can make use of it. It is an empathy based on a fundamental trust that the other person will be there for me when I need him or her and that I also will be there for the other person. It is, however, an intimacy that is based on expectations about what an effort we will both make and the risk taking and the acceptance of anxiety that will occur. Part of my role as a therapist is to expect strengths of my clients, and I am rarely disappointed. Perhaps that was the other reason that the client with the desolate dream shocked me so much. I had assumed that capacity for empathy in her and her dream suggested that it was not available.

It is crucial that our *contributions to therapy be clear and coherent.* The need for clarity first arises because of the important role of feedback from the therapist during therapeutic reconstruction. Validation and invalidation are crucial tools in the therapy process. Therefore, if feedback to clients about their construing is not provided clearly, the desired validation and invalidation will not occur (Leitner & Guthrie, 1993). This can be seen in my therapy with Christine, when, if she had not been able to understand the intended meaning of my statements to her, then she may not have begun to reconstrue in the way she did. Also, moving from individual constructs to more embracing stories, they too need to be clear. If the stories we tell in therapy are not clear they will not help in reconstruction. Our stories, however, need to be coherent, credible, and useful as well. They need be internally consistent, believable, and provide a range of viable choices for our clients. This was apparent as Frank and I worked together. It was only when we both came to recognize the incoherence and constriction inherent in Frank's story that I was able to develop an alternative story for him that was coherent and provided a wider range of choices for him. This new story also needed to be credible to both Frank and me.

Therapist Goals and Strategies

It is also important to be aware of the contribution made to therapy by our own *goals and strategies,* which are also often influenced by earlier life experiences. Recognizing, and if necessary renegotiating, the goals toward which I find myself working is sometimes necessary. With Frank, for example, I found myself trying to reduce his anger. Yet, when I reflected on this intention of mine, I realized that Frank had many good reasons for that anger, only some of which were available to us to work on in therapy. I also reminded myself that, when I worked in my own therapy on my own expression of anger, I saw it as powerfully destructive. I believed, I found, that my anger had killed several of the men in my life, including my father. It was only by testing the effects of this anger on my long-suffering therapist that I came to see it as somewhat less powerful. Frank's intense anger would, I believe, have been frightening to many others but to me it had an especially powerful quality. I therefore needed to move away from approaching that goal directly with Frank to retell his story so as to reduce the current sources of anger in his life.

A strategy that therapists can use with some success in therapy is humor. Personal construct therapists have been urged to be playful in therapy and to let go of current interpretations of both therapists and clients in this way (Epting, 1981). Humor can become an integral part of the intimate relationship between therapist and client so that gentle invalidation of my client's construing can be carried out through jokes made originally by either the therapist or the client. Ethel had her "Annie Get Your Walking Stick" joke, which for many sessions after she first ventured it served as a cheerful and yet useful reminder to us both that her stories needed to be based on a realistic assessment of her growing physical frailty.

Supervision of Therapists

Supervision from other experienced therapists of our contribution to therapy is essential. Like therapy, supervision occurs between meaning-making and validation-seeking people who bring to supervision their own construct systems. It, too, involves transference because the constructs that we use in therapy and supervision have always been used by us before. My primary task as a personal construct therapist in supervision is not to learn new therapeutic techniques but to understand and extend the ways in which I, as the therapist in supervision, make sense of my clients (Kenny, 1988). In such supervision, I come to ask better questions about myself and my clients. I can also try to come to terms with the cognitive and emotional demands of being a constructivist therapist (Mahoney, 1995).

Such supervision usually takes place in groups of therapists in a general climate of validation. Therapists in supervision are encouraged to be aware of our own dependencies or whom we see as providing us with help. It is also helpful for us to make summaries of the therapy, evaluate what occurs, and take risks as therapists. Summaries of therapy sessions are made at two levels in some supervision of this constructivist kind: (a) a concrete account of what occurred and (b) a more abstract account at the level of ideas from personal construct therapy (Kenny, 1988). As if is important in supervision too because therapists in supervision may need to behave, believe, and feel as if we were our clients in order to understand how those clients are construing events.

LEARNING FROM CLIENTS

One of the aspects of therapy that I most enjoy is that I learn so much from my clients. This is possible because they let me into their private inner worlds. I learn about their courage and many other strengths, as well as their capacity to use humor even when dealing with disability and death. I learned so much from two very different clients, my relationships with whom I have described in some detail in this book. Frank was not an easy client for me because of his intense anger. Yet, he taught me much by his acceptance of that anger and the confusion that went with it. Because of this I have become more able to accept such anger and confusion in other clients and also, from time to time, in myself. The other client whom I would mention here is Ethel who taught me about wisdom. Her ability to accept her own physical frailty and yet still maintain her stories about herself as an integrated being with continuity and her developing sense of oneness with others were striking. She also became more able to acknowledge the contributions of herself and others and to acknowledge their worth. I hope to be able to manage some of this myself at her age if I am fortunate enough to live so long.

BEING AN EFFECTIVE PERSONAL CONSTRUCT THERAPIST

How to become a more effective personal construct therapist involves therapists in coming to understand our own construing, especially through our own therapy, monitoring our own ethical position, and being aware of our contributions to therapy, especially through supervision. This process of becoming a better therapist is best carried out using the ideas of personal construct therapy, as I have described them in this book. These ideas include viewing reality as a constructed representation and taking a subjective perspective with clients. The view of therapy that is presented here is of therapy as being about meanings and stories, with both therapists and clients as construers. Joint reconstruction then becomes the key process in therapy. This therapy then involves the strategies of goal setting, storytelling, and a range of special techniques for understanding and helping clients. The focus of this therapy is historical and on psychological processes rather than on problems. When these ideas of personal construct therapy are used to understand ourselves and our clients, it becomes possible to conduct effective therapy as well as learn much from our clients.

Personal construct therapy has some unique qualities. My account of it has treated therapists in the same way that it has clients because this approach is reflexive. This means that the goals of both clients and therapists are considered, as are their ways of making sense of change. The metaphors both of us use to guide our lives are also included in therapy. However, the major contribution of this approach has been, I believe, in the view it offers of clients and therapists as tellers of stories, with therapy providing the main opportunity for clients to retell theirs.

This is my answer to that question that I asked earlier: "But how do you do therapy?" In my answer, I hope I have succeeded in filling in some more parts of a story of the reconstructive process of change. Of course, my story, even if it is a more consistent and coherent story than it was before I wrote this book, is only one of the many alternative stories that we can use to make sense of our clients and ourselves.

READINGS

Self-Monitoring of the Construing of the Therapist

Cohen, C.D., & Cooley, S. (1983). Psychological training programs for direct services to the ageing. *Professional Psychology, 14,* 720–728.

Epting, F. (1984). *Personal construct counselling and therapy.* Chichester: Wiley.

Gatz, M., & Pearson, C.E. (1988). Ageism revisited and the provision of psychological services. *American Psychologist, 43,* 184–188.

Kelly, G.A. (1955). *The psychology of personal constructs.* New York: Norton.

Kenny, V. (1987). Autopoesis and alternativism in psychotherapy: Fluctuations and reconstructions. In F. Fransella & L. Thomas (Eds.), *Experimenting with personal construct psychology.* London: Routledge & Kegan Paul.*

Kenny, V. (1988). Changing conversations: A constructivist model of training for psychotherapists. In G. Dunnett (Ed.), *Working with people: Clinical uses of personal construct psychology.* London: Routledge.*

Rabbitt, P., & Abson, J. (1991). Do older people know how good they are? *British Journal of Psychology, 82,* 132–151.

Viney, L.L. (1993). *Life stories: Personal construct therapy for the elderly.* Chichester: Wiley.

Self-Monitoring the Ethical Position of the Therapist

Bannister, D. (1983). The internal politics of psychotherapy. In D. Pilgrim (Ed.), *Psychology and psychotherapy.* London: Routledge & Kegan Paul.*

Beauchamp, T.L., & Childress, J.T. (1983). *Principles of biomedical ethics.* New York: Oxford.

---

* Most useful readings.

Dardenne, P., & Mahtani, A. (1989). *Transcultural counselling in action*. London: Sage.
Fairbairn, S., & Fairbairn, G. (1987). *Psychology, ethics and change*. London: Routledge & Kegan Paul.
Gilligan, C. (1982). *In a different voice*. Cambridge MA: Harvard University Press.
Gray, L.A., & Harding, A.K. (1988). Confidentiality limits with clients who have the AIDS virus. *Journal of Counselling and Development, 66,* 219–223.
Kain, C.D. (1988). To breach or not breach: Is that the question? A response to Gray and Harding. *Journal of Counselling and Development, 68,* 224–225.
Lakin, M. (1991). *Coping with ethical dilemmas in psychotherapy.* Elmsford, NY: Pergamon.
Lawless, D.J. (1989). Religious values in the workplace. *Organisational Development Journal, 11,* 1–9.
Mental Health Task Force. (1991). *Mental health: A statement of rights and responsibilities.* Canberra: Australian Government Printing Service.
Pope, K.S. (1990). Therapist–patient sexual involvement: A review of the research. *Clinical Psychology Review, 10,* 477–490.*
Ross, M.W. (1989). Psychosocial ethical aspects of AIDS. *Journal of Medical Ethics, 15,* 74–81.
Sue, D.W. (1981). *Counselling the culturally different.* New York: Wiley.
Steiner, M., Newall, J.D., & Garcia, C.T. (1984). *Ethical issues in psychology.* New York: Dorsey.
World Health Organization. (1981). *Global strategy for health for all by the year 2000.* Geneva: Author.

Self-Monitoring the Contributions to Therapy of the Therapist

Epting, F. (1981). An appraisal of personal construct psychotherapy. In H. Bonarius, R. Holland, & S. Rosenberg (Eds.), *Personal construct psychology—Recent advances in theory and practice.* London: Macmillan.*
Kalekin-Fischmann, D., & Walker, B. (1995). *The construction of group realities: Culture, society and personal construct theory.* Melbourne, FL: Krieger.
Leitner, L., & Guthrie, A.J. (1993). Validation of therapist interventions in psychotherapy: Clarity ambiguity and subjectivity. *International Journal of Personal Construct Psychology, 6,* 281–294.
Mahoney, M.J. (1995). The psychological demands of being a constructivist therapist. In R.A. Neimeyer & R.J. Mahoney (Eds.), *Constructivism in Psychotherapy.* Washington, D.C.: American Psychological Association.

EXERCISES

1. Identify an interaction that you had with a client during which you felt anxious. What occurred in therapy to extend your construct

system beyond your range of convenience? (This exercise can also be carried out using the emotions of guilt and anger with their constructivist definitions.)

2. Identify an interaction that you had with a client in which your construing of intimate relationships was threatened.
3. Identify an interaction you had with a client during which you felt contentment and pleasure. Which of your constructs were confirmed? Were they constructs you use to make your work meaningful as a therapist?
4. Write two accounts of a single experience of therapy with a client. The first should be a concrete account of events and the second should be at a more abstract level using ideas from personal construct therapy.
5. Identify a client of yours whose actions you could not easily understand. Try behaving like that client in those ways. What constructs do you find yourself using? Do they help you to understand the constructs of your client?

APPENDIX:

THREE ACCOUNTS OF PERSONAL CONSTRUCT THERAPY*

---

* I am grateful that Ann Brassil, Barry McNamara, and Stephen Scicluna agreed to share their accounts of some personal construct therapy, written when they were therapists in training. These accounts, together with my brief comments on them, show something of the variety of ways in which therapists can make sense of and work with their clients.

"Life Sucks"

Ann Brassil

Name of Client: **Jamie**
Age: **19**
Referred by: **Department of Probation and Parole**

REASON FOR REFERRAL

Jamie was said by the probation officer to have a long history of stealing and other offenses and wanted help both to find out why he constantly stole and to learn ways to stop stealing. He had been recently charged with "goods in custody" (car seats and stereo) and "malicious damage" (smashed car window) and the court hearing was scheduled for 2 months later. Jamie was said to be genuine in his desire for counseling and knew that, although he had a court case pending, a court report may not be written.

PRESENTING PROBLEM

Jamie complained during the initial interview that he could not stop himself from "pinching stuff." Jamie described a history of being in trouble with the law since the age of 9 years old for offenses such as stealing, breaking and entering, and being an "uncontrollable child." Over recent years, Jamie said he had mainly been stealing cars or car accessories (e.g., car stereos, seats): He stole cars to go joyriding. Jamie said he wanted to stop stealing as he did not want to return to jail, both because he hated losing his freedom and because his past incarcerations had hurt his mother a great deal.

SPECIFIC PROBLEM AREAS IDENTIFIED DURING ASSESSMENT

Although Jamie initially asked for help in understanding why he stole and to learn ways to stop stealing, it soon became apparent in our discussions that there were a range of problem areas in Jamie's life. Some that we jointly identified included:

1. His stealing behavior.
2. His alcohol consumption.
3. His "transport" problems, especially his driving too fast.
4. His relationships with others, especially intimate relationships with women.
5. His control of his temper.
6. His negative attitude to life ("life sucks").
7. His self-esteem.

It became clear that underlying these problem areas were a range of dysfunctional beliefs and feelings by which Jamie had been organizing his life. Given that Jamie was experiencing significant difficulty leading a happy and satisfying life, identifying and changing these dysfunctional constructs of Jamie's became the focus of therapy.

THERAPY AND THE OFFENDING CONSTRUCTS

Preamble

Therapy began at the outset of our contact when we both attempted to come to a joint understanding of the reasons for Jamie's referral to me. Together we looked at Jamie's expectations that therapy would be a means of learning to change his dysfunctional behavior and a way of proving to a magistrate at a later court hearing that Jamie was serious about changing his aberrant ways. We also arrived at some understanding of my role as a coevaluator of Jamie's problems rather than Jamie seeing me as someone who "would fix him." A therapeutic contract of six sessions was initially agreed on and later extended at

Jamie's request (albeit expressed rather ambivalently at that stage due to his continuing difficulty in making positive decisions about his welfare). Therapy continues at the time of this writing and the first 10 sessions are the basis of this report. Jamie is seen as a long-term psychotherapy client at this stage.

One of the purposes of therapy with Jamie was to improve his understanding of and ability to deal with the problems in his life that were limiting his optimal level of functioning and thereby increasing the chances that he commit illegal offenses and be sent to jail. Together we hoped to integrate Jamie's self in his world more successfully. Although this was an aim that Jamie and I shared, it was very difficult for Jamie to articulate this due to his very restricted use of language. This seemed to stem from a combination of factors including his poor education, his emotional defensiveness, and his lack of "psychological mindedness." I found myself very often searching for the words for Jamie to describe what he was trying to say rather than waiting for him to express himself in his own fashion, although I did this by incorporating Jamie's own language, metaphors, and style of relating and extending this when the opportunity arose as much as possible. A goal I then imposed in therapy was that of extending Jamie's language skills to aid his ability to understand and express himself.

As therapy progressed, it became a more comfortably constructive dialogue between Jamie and myself in which the purpose of our time together was to elaborate and expand Jamie's construct system (my language, not his). We worked toward achieving the personal changes he sought by increasing the range of his construct system and identifying areas of conflict between his constructs in order to integrate these more meaningfully. Adopting an open approach, the tone of the interactions between Jamie and me was largely conversational as we both attempted to make sense of his meanings and understandings and challenge these where necessary. Rapport between Jamie and myself improved steadily and this was based on a number of factors. Not to be underestimated was the fact that I came to like Jamie and this provided important validation for Jamie to see himself as a worthwhile person.

Humor was used throughout as an important therapeutic device. By making light of some issues, it was possible to loosen Jamie's (at times) very tight construing, allowing the necessary expansion and change to his construct system. Humor also served to break down the therapist–client boundary, helping Jamie to challenge more comfortably and confront my interpretations of his meanings. In this way, we were able to come to a better understanding of Jamie's feelings and beliefs. Thus, it also served as a constant barometer as to whether I was suspending my own construct system in coming to understand and subsume Jamie's.

Jamie's Depressive Construing

As my work with Jamie progressed, it became clear that Jamie's core construing was pervasively depressive. This was evident in many ways. There was an obvious lack of interpersonal construing and associated conflicting relationships, as well as his maintaining a great self–other distance. He showed a general lack of construing in the realm of personal feelings and an overriding tendency to use only the negative pole of his constructs or to use markedly polarized construing (all or nothing) and only engage in slot changing in his views about issues or people. His negative, core role structure was evidenced by his negative constructions about himself and his constant self-devaluation. He believed himself to be unintelligent, unable to control his behavior, incapable of making decisions about his behavior, and troubled by personal meaninglessness. It was as if the only major validation he gained was about his superordinate and largely impermeable construction that he was not in charge of his life or intrinsically entitled to a positive future. From our discussions, it appeared that this constricted construing of Jamie's was probably developed as a way of reducing further invalidation of his cherished identities in relation to others, of his core role construing. This suggested to me that Jamie, however dysfunctionally, was trying to create meaning in his life, to "make sense of" his own existence but required assistance in loosening and expanding his construct system.

The alteration to Jamie's depressive construing became the central goal of therapy. To this end, a broad range of therapeutic techniques were utilized. Some of these were deliberately chosen as useful "loosening" devices and included humor, as already mentioned, experimentation with choices, and personal decision making. There was also much reality testing, cognitive restructuring to help him compete with his belief system about himself, increasing the variety and number of positive experiences Jamie engaged in, and validating his negative life experiences, whereas at the same time helping him develop alternative interpretations of events and ways of dealing with the same. I also used praise of his achievements in therapy wherever possible and genuine uncritical acceptance of Jamie as a person and as a construer in difficulties, together with exploring the positive poles of some of his constructs.

When Jamie's dysfunctional constructs had undergone sufficient dilation to allow the inclusion of new experiences and new elements into his construing, the process of reconstruction began. This involved challenging some of Jamie's beliefs and being more confrontational with Jamie's negative interpretations of events (our discussions in fact became quite heated at times), much use of casual enactments and fixed-role therapy to provide experiences just outside the range of Jamie's construct system (as a test of possible new constructions about events for Jamie), and to test the predictive validity of the alternative stories he was developing. Much of the work done by Jamie was carried out outside the therapeutic relationship in which he tested his new constructions in the "real" world.

Thinking Versus Feeling

Jamie experienced a great deal of difficulty in relation to his emotions. He said he felt totally overwhelmed by his feelings, such that he felt incapable of stopping himself reacting if his emotional response was sufficiently intense. He was, at the outset of therapy, adamant that if "temptation" came he was helpless to stop himself doing what it was so tempting to do. His recent means of managing his problems was in line with his then construction of himself as being out of control; that is, he avoided temptation at all costs. To do this, he had been staying at home all the time when not engaged in "legitimate" activities, such as visiting his probation and parole officer, solicitor, or myself. I got the impression of somebody who felt compelled to separate himself from society so that he could see no temptation, hear no temptation, and feel no temptation. The fact that giving in to temptation was such an issue for Jamie was also indicative of his depressive state: In the absence of sufficient positive experiences, Jamie engaged, albeit unconsciously, in vicarious thrill or pleasure-seeking activities.

This feeling of subservience to his emotions pervaded many facets of Jamie's life and was intrinsically bound up with his stealing behavior, his excessive alcohol consumption, his driving too fast and dangerously, and his, at times, lack of control over his temper (this is discussed later in relation to his brother Glenn). Therapy therefore was aimed at understanding and then loosening and expanding the range of a number of dysfunctional, and at times, related constructions he held about himself. These included constructs about being unable to control his behavior when his emotions were involved, about his heart ruling his head (his feelings overriding his thinking), about his being helpless in the face of (irresistible) temptation versus having the freedom to make choices and decisions about his behavior, and about his right to expect and engineer a happy life versus accepting everything as being determined the overridingly negative. When this project was under way, it was then hoped to reintegrate new and more constructive beliefs such that he felt able to function more positively. Management of each of the aforementioned problem areas are briefly discussed.

Stealing. Jamie was encouraged to see himself as being able to master the temptation to steal cars when it arose rather than having to avoid having everything to do with cars (including looking at cars when walking down the street). We called this "facing temptation." Jamie was very reluctant to do this when we explored it as one of a range of options because it conflicted with his established construct about temptation being irresistible. We entered into some debate about the need to develop alternative behaviors, despite the fact that Jamie's avoidance behaviors worked to keep him out of trouble with the law at the present time. By the process of pyramiding his ideas, Jamie came to a new understanding of his problem as not being related solely to the existence of cars and their intrinsic appeal but to his feelings of not being in charge of his behavior and, at a more superordinate level of construction, his life. Introducing the notion of "choosing not to steal," Jamie was encouraged to see himself as in control of his behavior and as able to make decisions about what he would or would not do in a given situation.

In the homework assignment between sessions, Jamie was encouraged to behave as if he was able to resist the temptation to steal cars. To do this, he was asked to initially put himself in a relatively "safe" situation with some tempting cars (e.g., outside a showroom of fast cars where he would be unlikely to be able to steal even if he wanted to). It was agreed he would stand and have a good look at these cars allowing himself to appreciate them for the qualities he obviously admired, rather than avoiding observing them due to the seductiveness of the dreaded temptation. He was also encouraged to engage in a range of positive self-statements about his ability to "look and not touch." Although Jamie said openly that he feared that "the temptation might be too great" and that he preferred the safer option of avoiding having anything to do with cars, he agreed to try this out.

Jamie reported back at the next session that he had been successful in that he had found out that he could "look but not touch," an extremely important revelation for Jamie and having vast implications for the onset of changes in his core constructions. Following much praise, encouragement, and discussion about useful tactics, Jamie said over the following sessions that he was becoming "a bit more confident about not stealing, that the way I think about what I do has changed" and later still that he felt he had changed a great deal as although he felt in some respects "the same as before, I just don't do the same things." Jamie said that one of the main changes he felt he had made was that before he "used to think about things but couldn't pull them all together" but now he was learning to do so, to make decisions, and to be in charge.

Alcohol. Like Jamie's difficulty with stealing, Jamie's problems with alcohol stemmed from his belief that once tempted he was incapable of curbing his behavior. When I first met Jamie he was "on the wagon" so to speak. He explained that if he consumed any quantity of alcohol then he was bound to become paralytically drunk and, at these times, he was more likely to commit criminal offenses. To avoid this, he felt he could not drink at all. Although this superficially appeared to be an ideal solution to his problems with alcohol, it certainly did not seem to me to be a realistic and lasting solution given the probable future influence of his culture and alcohol-consuming peer group.

Given his success with controlling his behavior in relation to stealing cars, it was suggested to Jamie that he may like to try an alternative to remaining sober or getting drunk, that being choosing the amount he would like to drink and then stopping once he had reached his limit. Jamie again professed reluctance to change his tried and true method, so it was left up to him which of these methods he would like to go on experimenting with. Within a few sessions, Jamie cockily announced that not only had he been to a party and socialized positively with others (see later section on interpersonal relationships) but had also monitored his level of intoxication during the entire evening (although this is not to say his drinking was moderate) and felt an increase in his newfound confidence about his self-control.

Driving ("Transport"). Jamie's difficulty with driving involved a number of his constructs. He said he felt unable to control the temptation to drive (or ride a motor bike) too fast just for the thrill of it but qualified this by asserting that this occurred only when he owned or, in the past, had stolen the vehicle in question. Jamie said he had no difficulty controlling his behavior if the vehicle belonged to someone he knew, although he was baffled as to the reasons for this distinction. Discussing this at length it became apparent that Jamie's difficulties lay in the interaction between his general tendency to behave impulsively, as discussed earlier, and his lack of apparent concern for his own well-being. This fell into the category of: "What's the sense in planning?", an issue that came up repeatedly in therapy for Jamie.

Working on Jamie's difficulties with "transport" (as he liked to call it) then became a metaphor for Jamie engaging positively in his life, for giving up his cherished and dysfunctional superordinate construct that "life sucks," and replacing it with the more constructive belief that he could choose behavior to make situations better or worse for himself. During our work together on this issue, we discussed and we digressed, and at times I found it difficult not to impose my personal constructions onto Jamie's experience. At one stage, I asked Jamie to engage in role reversal with me as a way of getting him to dilate his constructions about what would constitute acceptable behavior for himself. By the 10th session, Jamie was considering buying a bike that would be the easiest to ride slowly because he wanted to remain out of trouble with the law. This was indicative of Jamie's changing attitude to himself in his world where he not only had begun to see himself as capable of controlling his behavior, but also was choosing courses of action that were most likely to lead to a good future for himself. This was a positive step indeed and a testimony to his growing sense of personal freedom.

Interpersonal Relationships

At the outset of therapy, Jamie tended to construe his relationships with others in a very constricted and often unipolar way. This was abundantly evident in his relationships with his family. He depicted his mother as a paragon of virtue, someone who could do no wrong and for whom he could not entertain a critical thought without this being a veritable betrayal. At the other extreme were his constructions of people he felt animosity for, including his father, brother Glenn, the police, and most of the rest of humanity. He saw these people as bad and destructive with not really an endearing quality.

Jamie's conversations about people he felt animosity for were tinged by a sense of guilt that he could not master himself sufficiently to deal constructively with these people. This guilt was indicative of an awareness (for Jamie at a very low level) of dislodgement of Jamie's self from his core role structure. I believe this dislodgement occurred in two areas. The first one related to Jamie having albeit submerged ideal expectations about people behaving in a nurturing way with each other and conflict arising in Jamie when this did not occur. The second related to Jamie's feeling that he may lose control of his temper when these people baited him, when he prided himself on being emotionally impervious. The hostility Jamie felt could be understood in terms of Jamie continuing to try to extort validational evidence about people's caring behavior, and about his own emotionlessness, even though both of these had proven to be untrue.

Therapy regarding Jamie's interpersonal relationships was aimed at changing his apparent method of dealing with conflict in his preferred construct pole by slot changing to the nonpreferred pole. Specifically, those constructs related to people being "good versus bad" and his behavior being "in control versus out of control" were expanded to allow him to conceptualize people's behavior as either good or bad and himself as making choices about his response to those behaviors of others. This was particularly pertinent in Jamie's learning to reconstrue his relationship with his brother Glenn. Jamie claimed he had in the past no alternative other than to use physical violence as a way of controlling Glenn's provocative and violent behavior. In therapy, Jamie began to reconstrue Glenn's behavior as a successful way of drawing attention to himself and Jamie's response to this as only one of a number of alternatives available to Jamie. As a consequence of this new understanding, Jamie reported feeling much more confident in his ability to make decisions about his behavior with Glenn and in general felt good about himself in the process (even though he has not as yet developed a sufficient repertoire of alternative behaviors to manage Glenn effectively and nonviolently).

When Jamie's relationships outside the family were discussed, his polarized construing was even more apparent. Jamie was not able to describe his feelings about, or his relationship with, these people and he depended on rather gross generalizations to categorize people and distance himself in relation to them. An example of this was in his attitude to the police whom he saw as being totally corrupt. (We all know this is not the case and I obviously had real trouble suspending my construct system regarding this matter.) Given that the police purportedly carry out the biddings of society at large, Jamie argued that society itself was fundamentally unjust and there was no way in which he could survive happily in such a system. Initially, at my suggestion, we both coined the phrase "what's the sense in planning" to describe this issue (although I knew it would be better described as "there is no sense in planning," I wanted to move Jamie from this impermeable superordinate construct to testing alternative constructions), and found it to underpin and perhaps be the foundation of Jamie's negative constructions about life. In therapy, this belief system was challenged in a number of ways. Jamie was asked to actively extend the range of positive activities and relationships he engaged in. Needless to say, this technique alone was almost impossible for Jamie, as it conflicted so totally with a superordinate construct (with a suspended positive pole) he held about not being able to attain happiness in his life. In the later stages of therapy, more time was given to examining and challenging this belief, determining positive projects for Jamie, and encouraging him to develop relationships based on common positive interests with people (e.g., working on cars) rather than just avoiding relationships due to his past association with people who encouraged his delinquent behavior. Learning that he could choose his friends was another important step in his feeling empowered to control his life and in his feeling he could increase the range of people he socialized with. He even found he could develop a friendship with a probationary police officer!

Related to this issue, at the outset of therapy Jamie seemed confused and vaguely disturbed about how to deal with women in his peer group. Jamie had had one steady girlfriend in the past but she had broken off the relationship by letter when he was in jail. Jamie said he was very hurt by this, that he "tried my best then she pissed me off." Jamie said that because he gets "too deeply involved too quick" and that because the only thing that makes him cry is "emotional stuff, not physical," he did not intend to get involved with women again. By avoiding close interpersonal relationships, Jamie felt that he could then let his head rule his heart, something he felt incapable of doing when he got involved with others, especially in romantic relationships. Here again was evidence of Jamie not feeling in control of his life, in this case of his emotional relationships, when individuals did not fit strictly into his tight construing of them as being trustworthy or untrustworthy.

In therapy, the issue of his relationships with women was addressed in a very practical way. Following discussions about what Jamie wanted from a relationship with a woman, he was encouraged to enter into relationships on the basis of friendship, as this was one of his main requirements. Previously conceptualizing himself as being either "in" or "out" of a romantic relationship, Jamie's construing became expanded to include different levels of emotional relating based on his choice about the particular person. He came to understand that his head and his heart could work together in his best interest rather than representing conflicting needs in himself. Of course, Jamie's progress in this area was very slow and he was only just feeling confident enough to experiment with his male and female relationships in the more recent sessions.

CONCLUSION

It is early, after only 12 sessions, to be drawing conclusions about the changes Jamie has made. So far, all the major issues identified as causing Jamie difficulty have been addressed in therapy, as have many other issues that cannot be recounted here due to space constraints. Jamie has been to court and has been let off this time with a bond and a moderate fine. Now is the time when it will become clear whether the changes he has made in therapy are of intrinsic value to him or not. He has had such a poor start to life and the culture from which he comes is certainly not conducive to a straight life. In his favor, he is bright (though undisciplined), sensitive to his own needs and the needs of others and, despite appearances, certainly is always looking for ways to overcome difficulties, even though he has not always found effective strategies by himself or from within his sociocultural milieu.

Countertransference? Perhaps a little, but I prefer to call it morals instead. This lad is at a crossroad in his life. He needs more than a passive therapeutic relationship or someone who is disinterested in his welfare. He needs to be actively engaged in therapy, to feel that he is of value in his own right and to be confronted when he is being provocative or is opting out both of which come naturally to him. Jamie needs to be encouraged to function at a personal level and for this reason the therapeutic relationship was particularly important for Jamie that changes could be made. In this way, therapy with Jamie truly did provide the testing ground from which he could then feel encouraged to test his new constructions in the real world. It was a bit of an honor for me that Jamie at one point said: "We are both Bankstown people," indicating the extent to which he felt he could relate to me.

What of personal construct therapy amid all this? I believe it was the intervention of choice. By being sensitive to the importance of my role as a validator of Jamie and by being keenly aware of the need to suspend my construct system while subsuming his, it was possible to create what I believed to be the ideal setting for therapeutic change for Jamie. This is not to say that I think this is necessarily the case for effective intervention with all clients. There certainly were times in therapy in which what I was doing had little relation to therapeutic reconstruction per se (e.g., discussing compensation claim procedures). However, using the therapeutic ethos of this psychotherapeutic approach, Jamie's experience of himself changed from being bound in his core role constructions to a depressive outlook on life to looking forward to ways to continue to create positive meaning in his life. At this stage, he has begun to develop a more complex, realistic, flexible, and integrated set of constructs for making sense of his experience and there is now a developing sense of self-confidence and self-worth in Jamie.

COMMENTS FROM LINDA VINEY

This account of personal construct therapy has a number of clear strengths. For example, therapist and client can be seen working together as they identify areas of possible therapeutic goals that they can have. This therapist shows genuine openness to her client, Jamie's construing, and uses his metaphors (e.g., his difficulties with transport); together they have retold some of his stories, for example, about temptation. The only therapeutic issue I would raise with this therapist concerns her apparent lack of recognition that some of his stories about his relationships with others were likely to be played out in therapy with her. Her self-monitoring is the other strength of this therapist. She has been aware that she has occasionally "imposed" goals on Jamie, such as his acquiring better language skills, and has wryly admitted her tendency to use her own stories to make sense of his experiences.

"I Can't Love That Baby as I Know I Should"

Barry McNamara

Name of Client:	Lauren
Age:	25
Referred by:	Dr. P. (Psychiatrist)
Reason for Referral:	Lauren had been diagnosed as suffering from postpartum depression.

EXPERIENCES OF PRESENTING CLIENT

Lauren's most notable problem was her inability to parent her 8-week-old son Guy. This inability extended to not coping with Guy's incessant crying and his perceived excessive demands on Lauren's time both day and night, her unwillingness to feed and look after Guy, and her overwhelming feeling of "I can't love that baby as I know I should." As a consequence, Lauren described herself as profoundly depressed and she had seriously considered suicide on two occasions in the past 3 weeks. She was currently taking antidepressant medication.

My initial contact with Lauren was in response to a referral for the crisis team, of which I was a member, to intervene by providing support for Lauren. We visited Lauren twice daily for 1 week, predominantly to monitor the condition of the baby and Lauren's potential for suicide. However, as the "crisis" ameliorated, I offered Lauren the opportunity for individual therapy as a means of coming to terms with her present difficulties.

Lauren was a 25-year-old attractive woman who was extremely distressed at the turn of events that had overcome her in recent weeks. She was genuinely devastated by her reaction to Guy: Never in a million years believing that she would react like this. This position was backed by her husband Steve who described Lauren as "the best prepared mother in this town." She had read every book on baby care she could lay her hands on, believing that this would prepare her for any problems and "haunted" the Baby Health Centre for additional information and reassurance (as a Baby Health sister was later to attest) prior to Guy's birth. However, nothing Lauren read or learned had helped her with her current feelings toward Guy. She felt "depressed, helpless, hopeless, and not in control."

LAUREN'S CONSTRUING

For Lauren, "depression" connoted a feeling of utter worthlessness brought about by invalidation of her core constructs. This invalidation was due to the fact that, although Lauren "had tried everything" to cajole and pacify Guy, he had not responded to her efforts. Consequently she had the overpowering sense that "he must hate me" and, by corollary, "I must be a bad mother." At these times, Lauren's response was that she usually clammed up not wishing to inflict herself or her misery on anyone. She did this by going to her bedroom, closing the door, going to bed, and refusing to speak with anyone. Such a state could persist from a matter of hours to several days, thus resulting in exacerbating her neglect of Guy.

This feeling of depression, however, was neither a recent nor birth-linked phenomenon. Lauren recalled that she had been periodically "low" since about 11 years old, "when I first started growing up and realizing I was becoming a woman." Lauren could not recall "the last time I felt really happy." Ironically, when she felt herself becoming too happy, Lauren then "became depressed" in an effort to avoid the inevitable "big drop" from happiness to despair. This coping strategy, she felt, related to her present predicament with Guy. Lauren said she was almost afraid to allow herself to become involved with Guy for fear of him subsequently rejecting her: "If I don't give too much then I won't get too hurt." This accounted for her attempting to distance herself from the baby by refusing to breast-feed him, pick him up, cuddle him, or initiate contact with him in general.

As these narratives evidence, Lauren's construing of her world could best be described as constricted. This was a way of coping by which Lauren endeavored to reduce the number of incompatible events with which she had to deal in an attempt to impose some semblance of order in her world. Lauren displayed characteristic "depressive" self-devaluation in the form of alternately, negative, or ambivalent self-construing. In other words, she was exacting negative rather than positive information from her ongoing experiences almost as if she was cognitively primed to selectively attend to negative information only. Another form of this cognitive rigidity, characteristic of polarized construing, was highlighted by Lauren's tendency to interpret events in her world in an all-or-nothing fashion without any shades of gray. Finally, she viewed herself as different from significant others, rejecting established stereotypes, in an effort to distance herself from significant others in her life.

EXPERIMENTING WITH EXPERIENCE

The key to assisting Lauren to cope with and overcome her present difficulties lay in encouraging her to experiment with extensions and revisions of her construct system so as to discover new and more effective ways of construing her world. In other words, the primary aim of therapy was to help her to be able to dilate her construct system.

I have chosen only a sample of the interventions that Lauren and I experimented with as an example of our attempts to reconstrue her view of the world. Because therapy has been extensive (currently 21 sessions), it was not possible to relate all of our attempts at reconstruing within the constraints of this report.

In an effort to mobilize Lauren out of her depressive mind-set, I thought it important to demonstrate to her that there were a variety of ways of viewing an event that may differ from a construct she superimposed on the event. To this end, I attempted to engage Lauren in an exercise exploring a creativity cycle with reference to the way in which she interpreted Guy's reaction toward herself. Lauren construed Guy's incessant crying and whining when she touched him or picked him up as indicating that "he hates me, I can see it in his eyes. But if I give him up now he won't hate me when he grows up." We selected this construct and set about generating alternative ways of interpreting Guy's reaction. Lauren, after some considerable encouragement, volunteered a variety of possible alternatives to explain Guy's behavior including that he was experiencing simple somatic disturbances (e.g., wind or colic), that he was not being held the right way, and that he did not have the "power to be able to think the thoughts" she attributed to him at this young age. From this we critically assessed each of these alternatives and eliminated the inappropriate ones. This enabled us to narrow down the choice to the fact that Guy was not, at this young age, capable of "thinking," that his whining and irritability was merely a baby's way of reacting to some distress.

This breakthrough of being able to reconstrue Guy's reaction gave Lauren immense relief and, more importantly, newfound hope. She remarked how she now felt able "to break out of the mold of seeing things only one way." This was a momentous step in therapy for us as it represented the first time Lauren had the strength to throw off the shackles of her depression and to embrace renewed hope. It also served to validate my role as an effective helper, something that I had been struggling to assert in employing this new approach to therapy. Thus, Lauren had greater confidence in me and was thus able to more readily trust me, a crucial step and turning point in our relationship.

So then, by providing Lauren with the alternative narrative that Guy's reaction to her was normal, I was able to invalidate some of Lauren's current peripheral construing and provide her with new information that she could use to reconstrue her experience and adopt a new course of action over which she could exercise control.

Another example of Lauren's constricted construing was evidenced in her observation that she was experiencing difficulty in fulfilling the stereotypic role of a woman and, furthermore, a mother as she perceived it. Lauren remarked that she felt more comfortable in the company of men and in being involved in such "masculine" occupations as car mechanics at which she apparently excelled. She abhorred the "typical gossip" that women as a group indulged in. However, she found that men did not accept her "as an individual" when she joined in their conversation as they "cleaned up their language when I'm around. I wish they would accept me as me rather than as a woman."

Our discussion centered around how Lauren construed the role and function of a woman in our society and particularly in the small town milieu in which she lived. I asked her, as a homework assignment, to develop a self-characterization of herself as seen through the eyes of her best friend as a way of garnering more about Lauren's construing of herself as a woman. This approach immediately met with difficulties because, characteristically (for depressives), Lauren claimed that there was no person who filled that role. This led to a discussion of Lauren's construing of friendship and how she felt she had never been allowed to have friends "because of my mother's jealousy that someone could be so important in my life."

Associated with her negative self-construing was Lauren's tremendous lack of self-confidence. When I queried her about this, she said she had a "very low opinion of her own ability to make decisions" and consistently deferred to Steve's greater (so she assumed) experience and knowledge. These feelings seemed to have their genesis with her mother who had "always dominated me even when I was a child. She even chose my friends for me. I suppose that's where I got this feeling from." Although this "avoidance strategy" (i.e., avoiding making a decision) helped her maintain her low self-concept, Lauren harbored a deep resentment that Steven now discounted her feelings when important decisions needed to be made. For example, because Steve contributed 75% of the deposit when they bought their house, he had drawn up in the ownership documents that he owned 75% of the house. He did not, however, seek Lauren's opinion on this move. This attitude served to constantly destabilize and undermine Lauren's confidence in herself, which she construed as indicative of her "worthlessness as a person."

To eradicate this spiral of negative self-construing, I (gently) confronted Lauren by challenging her to demonstrate her construct system's internal consistency. On the one hand she was saying to Steve "you make the decisions because I am not worthy," whereas on the other she was upset because he now discounted her when decisions were made. When confronted with this dichotomy, Lauren realized that she was, albeit unknowingly, causing her own problem. To reconstrue this situation, we decided to jointly design an experiment using the technique of enactment that would center around developing a new, more assertive Lauren. In a series of graded steps not unlike systematic desensitization, we role played various situations in which Lauren would normally have said nothing at the time but later fumed over how she was not consulted. Lauren developed alternative narratives to her usual mode of response and, after practice using the gestalt "two-chair" technique, she was assigned the task of putting into practice these new strategies with Steve.

This approach had immediate effects. Steve was at first taken unawares by the "new," more assertive Lauren. However, as he later attested, he developed a new admiration for his wife whom he had now come to regard as an equal partner, something he had always wanted but felt unsure of encouraging Lauren to try because he felt she wanted him "to play the role of the protective, macho male."

At this point, it was clear that progress in therapy was being hindered by not having Steve available. Thus, Lauren and I decided to invite him to join in with us. Lauren had thought that he would be reluctant to do this, as he was a "shy, retiring type who does not talk about his feelings." However, Steve leapt at the opportunity and all subsequent therapy sessions have included him. As a consequence, we feel our sessions have been much more successful.

After several more sessions, we mutually decided to suspend therapy so as to give Lauren and Steve a chance to put into practice what had been discussed in the recent sessions. I did not hear from them for some time but did, however, call in on them when driving past one day. They seemed much more relaxed with each other and Lauren was holding Guy, a breakthrough in itself. We decided that Lauren would instigate when therapy should resume.

I received a phone call from Lauren several weeks ago to report that she was now feeling much happier with herself as a person. She was now able to assert herself and she and Steve were "getting on much better." However, she felt she was now ready to move on to deal with her feelings toward Guy, which "had improved but only slightly." She felt confident that, given the "success" of the previous therapy that she could overcome this problem also. We are currently involved in these issues.

POSTSCRIPT OR "HINDSIGHT IS A WONDERFUL THING"

There were, undoubtedly, significant errors committed by me during the course of therapy. Most of these were associated with my inexperience with this particular approach to therapy. Commonly, the most predominant error was an overly vigorous search for constructs, particularly in the early stages of therapy. At these times, I fear that I became overly involved in the theory and consequently inattentive to the practice.

An example of this situation is evidenced by Lauren's severe lack of confidence in the practical matters of parenting Guy, such as bathing, holding, feeding, and so forth. I chose to pursue the meaning of this inadequate parenting rather than listen to what she was telling me that she wanted practical assistance. Only when I arranged for a Baby Health sister to visit and advise Lauren on these basic matters was she prepared to join with me in pursuing therapy. However, my initial insensitivity lost me crucial "points" with Lauren that took some significant effort to recoup.

My initial decision not to employ a Repertory Grid with Lauren because she was not (in my initial opinion) appropriately psychologically minded was, in fact, incorrect. I feel we could have achieved more in a shorter amount of time if I had done this. I also failed to understand ways of working with some constructs once they were elicited.

However, the most disconcerting feeling for me, particularly early on in therapy, was that I did not feel we were making sufficient progress. This pervasive feeling was mirrored constantly (or perhaps initiated) by Lauren, who continually asked whether she was getting better yet or alternately that she did not think the therapy was working. I found myself reassuring her that "these things take time" but inwardly I was anguishing about "losing" this client (i.e., her confidence in me). I do not think I handled the situation well at that time.

COMMENTS FROM LINDA VINEY

This therapist has identified the interlocking stories that have trapped his client, Lauren, into her actions with her son Guy. He has also helped her to develop alternative stories about Guy's actions, which have given her a wider range of choices for her response to him. However, as with the first of these three therapeutic accounts, there has been no recognition that the client's interpersonal stories are likely to be replayed in transference. Also, there is a tendency for this therapist to identify therapeutic projects without consultation with Lauren, which results in a less than optimal therapeutic relationship . However, again in this account there is good evidence of self-monitoring by the therapist. He is critical of his own concern with theory to the exclusion of effective practice and aware of his own goal about maintaining his client's confidence in him.

"Burrowing Into Work"

Stephen Scicluna

Name of Client: Tony
Age: 46
Occupation: Builder
Marital Status: Divorced
Referred by: Self

REASON FOR REFERRAL

Tony phoned my center complaining of stress-related problems and an inability to relax. He said that he was engulfed by work, working up to 20 hr a day. Tony explained how on New Year's Eve he drank too much, and hit his lady. Consequently, he has a restraining order on him, he lives alone, and has little else apart from work.

TONY'S CONSTRUING

Tony's presenting complaint was that he was working too much and unable to relax. He believed that this had commenced when he accepted a more demanding position last year. He also hypothesized that his working long hours and inablility to relax were compounded by problems he was having with his ex-wife Julie with whom he was again having a relationship.

Tony identified as the precipitant to seeking therapy his becoming violent toward Julie following a New Year's Eve dinner at which he drank excessively. Tony's experience of drinking was "everything comes out—I don't think I should really drink. But then again it showed me that there is a lot bottled up." It seems that Tony construed himself as having personal issues that needed to be understood. His present level of construing was unsatisfactory and did not provide for suitable action.

Tony dealt with the problems he and Julie were having by dismissing them and attempting to organize a vacation for the two of them. He construed the main problem as being that they both needed "to escape," Tony from work and Julie from her interfering and influential family. However, Julie refused his offers to escape or in some way undermined them. In return, Tony would react by working longer hours, this compounded the stress experienced personally and within their relationship.

Tony construed this pattern as Julie not giving the relationship a chance. He described it accurately as a "dog chasing its tail" but was not aware of the more abstract psychological issues involved. He also admitted to not knowing how to break the cycle. The breaking point came while finally on vacation together: Tony's expectation of the relationship being improved was invalidated. Having his self-control diminished by alcohol and construing that he had little control over his relationship, Tony acted aggressively.

THERAPIST'S CONSTRUING

Tony impressed me as a very competent, business-like person. He seemed constrained in his ability to communicate on an emotional level, preferring to relay events in a factual manner without describing his feelings.

Tony's experience of drinking as previously described and the long time (4 months) between the event he identified as precipitating therapy and when he presented himself for therapy, suggested to me that Tony was ambivalent as to whether he wanted to understand what was happening to him, particularly his construing of his relationship with Julie.

I thought that Tony, although aware of the destructive pattern of events which had been repeated many times during the previous 12 months, was not aware of the more abstract, psychological issues that underlay them. One of the goals of therapy was to identify these issues and to bring them to Tony's awareness and understanding so that he could change his actions accordingly. Through understanding his construing, Tony would be able to integrate his cognitions with his emotions.

NEW WAYS OF CONSTRUING THROUGH NEW STORIES

Psychotherapy is successful only when both participants are ready to develop new stories. I felt that Tony needed to develop new stories about his relationship with Julie and about his work. However, I was unsure as to whether he was ready to develop new narratives, particularly about his relationship. For me, developing new stories about Tony was not difficult. However, I found presenting Tony with a new story about his relationship in a way that he would accept it exceedingly difficult. On the contrary and somewhat surprisingly, developing a new story about work occurred almost spontaneously as we explored his relationship. Tony's relationship with Julie and his work were the focus of therapy.

NEW STORIES ABOUT WORK

A large part of Tony's presenting problem was his inablility to limit the hours he spent working. He described waking at 5 a.m. and leaving for work by 6 a.m. His job involved traveling between numerous construction sites supervising and troubleshooting projects. On returning home at about 9 p.m., he would soon find himself assessing plans until late at night. Tony explained that although he wished to be able to limit his working hours, he had construed it as necessary given that he was on probation for 6 months, during which time he had to prove himself to his employer.

As therapy progressed, Tony began to spontaneously elaborate his construing about work. As he did, his story about work changed. Being on probation was no longer an adequate reason for working so hard, especially because the probationary period had already ended with Tony securing the position and receiving a substantial bonus. Trying to understand his construing about work, Tony said:

> "I have a problem being able to . . . I don't know whether its a guilt complex that I work so much, I'm certainly not trying to build an ego, I think its very important for me to achieve something right. Over the years of bankruptcies, monetary worries, et cetera, I have a huge desire to stabilize."

In our second session, Tony described his briefcase full of files that he took home every night as his "security rug." He compared himself to Linus the cartoon character who drags his blanket around behind him everywhere he goes. Tony then said that he was going to buy a slimmer briefcase and only carry two files. I praised this decision and encouraged Tony to search for other ways he could limit his working hours. It seemed that by being able to understand his construing better, Tony no longer needed such a big security rug.

Trying to help Tony reconstrue his working so hard, I asked him how he thought it fitted in with what was happening between Julie and himself. We soon found ourselves discussing a vicious circle in which Tony would attempt "escape" from work and the "situational" (e.g., familial problems) with Julie by arranging a vacation. Julie would respond by refusing or undermining the holiday, sometimes directly asking Tony to work on her house instead. Feeling rejected, Tony would set his plans aside and work harder. Consequently, Tony would get more tired, irritable, forgetful, and disoriented. The cycle would start again in hope of having a rest and perhaps a reprieve of their relationship.

Promoting this cycle was Tony's reaction to the emotional experience of having this relationship curtailed. In personal construct terms, Tony was experiencing a chronic sense of emptiness because his core role was being deprived of the validation that follows from meaningful involvement with others.

Tony responded to this situation by constriction or drawing in outer boundaries of his perceptual field by absorbing himself in his work. In this way, he retained the ability to anticipate experiences by restricting the events to be interpreted. This led Tony to a cycle of constriction and personal isolation. The more he constricted, the more isolated he became and the fewer people he had to interact with, as well as the less often he encountered events that invalidated his construing and forced a revision of his constricted system.

In our final session, Tony described himself as "burrowing into work" and "driving down a narrow channel." I viewed these descriptions as a useful confirmation of my constructions about Tony. Although they also reflected Tony's engineering background, they indicated that some reconstruing had taken place and work was now reconstrued as being an escape.

Changes in Tony's construing of work lead to some changes in action. He went out and bought himself a slimmer briefcase. He also came in for an appointment one morning looking notably relaxed and wearing a sweat suit. He explained that he had been up for most of the night caring for his ill mother and so was not prepared to go to work at the usual, early time. At one time, Tony said, feeling guilty would have prevented him from doing that.

When confronted with interpersonal events that lie beyond the range of their undeveloped systems of social construing, some people experience anxiety. Contrary to my initial construing of Tony's experience, he was not experiencing anxiety. Perhaps anxiety was minimal because Tony lacked an abstract, psychological approach to his relationship, viewing Julie in more concrete and egocentric terms. When Tony was confronted with an event that did lie beyond his range, he construed it as lacking control and reacted with violence.

NEW STORIES ABOUT HIS RELATIONSHIP

Individuals depend on others to validate their senses of identity. When close relationships are severed by divorce or death, individuals experience a partial disintegration of the self. Tony was on several occasions threatened with the possibility of rejection and separation and hence a partial disintegration of his self. Unfortunately, this was something that Tony had experienced several times in the past and was now trying dearly to avoid. Consequently, Tony was not willing to revise his constructions about Julie despite overwhelming evidence that she no longer wished to have anything to do with him.

Not willing to revise constructions to fit new experience, Tony was left with three choices: (a) to discount the invalidations and recast the same social "experiment" (try again), (b) selectively attend to only those events that are consistent with the original belief (constriction), or (c) force the other person to act in a manner consistent with these beliefs ("with hostility"). Tony seemed to make use of both discounting invalidations and constriction.

Tony initially dismissed Julie's refusal to go away on holidays and relabeled his request as selfishness on his part. Further invalidation occurred when Julie contracted genital herpes when on vacation alone. This too was dismissed by Tony, but was the beginning of him starting to doubt her.

By repeatedly dismissing Julie's invalidations, Tony opened the way for him to try again. He did this by organizing more vacations, working harder on Julie's house, buying her a sports car, and generally "just trying to please her." Despite his efforts, Julie remained "not responsive" and Tony "couldn't work it out." I conceptualized this as Tony experiencing a vague bewilderment as the peripheral and disjointed constructions by which he tried to construe Julie's motives and his behavior had to shift to accommodate repeated invalidation. Tony discounted Julie's actions, explaining that "She is going out of her way to be cruel. . . . I know Julie pretty well . . . its a facade . . . its a shame. . . . she has promised her family not to speak to me."

It was difficult for Tony to selectively attend to those events that were consistent with his construing because there was so few of them. To do so, he reached further back into the relationship, explaining that they had three or four separations in the past but had reconciled after each one.

I attempted to help Tony revise his constructions about his relationship with Julie. Believing that his constructions were void of sufficient feeling, I asked questions that focused on feelings not only of how events made him feel, but also to speculate on how they made Julie feel. To facilitate this process, I attempted to introduce words that classified and elaborated his emotions. I also asked Tony how various events fitted into his story about his relationship. This I hoped would force him to elaborate his story or at least identify areas that needed a lot more reconstruing, thus making him aware of its limitations.

At a later stage in therapy, when I thought I understood Tony's construing, I attempted to invalidate it by providing an alternative story. For example, I suggested that maybe this time Julie really meant it but that it would be difficult for him to accept that because to do so would probably mean acknowledging a separation that to him meant yet another "failure." I also suggested that being in a relationship meant stability for Tony and in his own words he had "a huge desire to stabilize."

Helping Tony reconstrue his relationship was one of the major projects of therapy. Unfortunately, I think it was only partially achieved. Although Tony's story was inadequate, mine was not sufficiently optimistic and so we did not agree on a new story.

Tony's story did not adequately cover Julie's behavior, consequently it did not provide for appropriate actions. At one point in our discussion, Tony attempted to justify his actions by suggesting that his behavior on one occasion was simple "good manners," and that he would have behaved like that toward any woman. I conceptualized this in terms of Tony's inability to construe Julie's construing and the limitation of his construing to provide suitable action. The content of Tony's story was also not specific enough to make predictions possible. When asked to predict in which direction the relationship would go, he could not hazard a guess. His narrative also failed to predict Julie's actions.

The alternative story that I presented did not provide Tony with actions that he was willing to take. It also predicted that the relationship would end. Thus, the outcome of my story was too pessimistic for Tony and he was not ready to accept it. My mistake was in developing such a story without sufficient input from Tony. Thus, it did not include enough of Tony's story. This error probably reflected my eagerness to do well with a new approach to therapy and the self-imposed time limit of five sessions. I also do not think I fully appreciated or respected Tony's construing, thus failing to be sufficiently accepting in my approach.

Tony needed to more accurately understand his construing. I could help this process once I understood his construing by helping him to integrate his cognitions with his emotions. As previously mentioned, I tried to do this by focusing on feelings and providing alternative stories, the latter with limited success. Greater advancement in understanding his construing occurred when we began to explore the concept of assertiveness.

TRYING TO UNDERSTAND HIS CONSTRUING

The idea to explore assertiveness came to me when Tony told me the story of his relationship with Julie. He described doing "things because she wanted it." Often, such things were quite outrageous and according to Tony "not my way of thinking." Tony also explained "I need to draw the line . . . need to learn to do that. . . . maybe that's my insecurity. . . . I'd like to put it down to caring for her. . . . maybe that's an excuse. . . . I don't know . . . it doesn't worry me that much." I construed Tony needing to "draw the line" as needing to be assertive. A little later in our discussion, Tony explained "if that makes her happy then all right. . . . What really gets me . . . if I go down that path . . . but then she wants more . . . then the line starts to go up, she calls me mean." Tony often felt that the message he was getting from Julie was: "Do what I want or I'll shoot off like a rocket."

Tony was given the following definition of assertiveness: A state of well-being that includes a sense of self-worth, a belief in our own rights and the rights of others, and the ability to communicate our rights effectively without denying the rights of others. This definition provided a foundation on which we could begin to build a more accurate construction of his construing to include cognitions and emotions.

For Tony, the opposite pole of being assertive was being easygoing. When asked what easygoing meant, he said that is how he wants to be in "personal relationships." He also equated easygoing with being in love and giving all he could to his partner. Thus, Tony's assertive/easygoing construct was a core construct that governed his identity within relationships. Asking Tony to describe Julie on the same construct revealed that he considered her as not caring about the feelings of others, being selfish, and hard to get on with.

To help Tony elaborate his construing I introduced the ideas of aggressive and passive styles of relating and suggested that we needed to distinguish between these and relating assertively. Initially, Tony found it difficult to distinguish between aggressiveness and assertiveness. However, after some discussion and examples, he moved on to describe himself as assertive at work and sometimes aggressive but passive in his relationship with Julie. He reconstrued Julie as aggressive.

A little later in our discussion, Tony explained that he could be assertive in his relationship with Julie but that he would be "frightened of losing her." Consequently, Tony explained "I backed down, looking back I was wrong, 'cause I lost a lot of respect." So then it seemed that Tony was beginning to integrate his cognitions with his emotions.

Tony was also starting to understand his construing and make more sense of his actions. With respect to feeling selfish for becoming violent, Tony said: "Now, looking back on it I don't feel so selfish, I'm starting to understand why I did it, I don't say that's right, but I do say that people have a breaking point and I reached it." Tony felt sorry for slapping Julie but now understood why he had done it.

Referring back to our definition of assertiveness, I asked Tony whether a belief in our own rights was the same as being selfish. After some thought he replied, "I think, in a relationship it could be . . . no, no, I. . . no, no we all have rights. . . . I have rights, no it's not being selfish when you think about it . . . it's not being selfish." Tony was now more willing to think and act assertively in relationships because to do so would no longer be construed as being selfish and in opposition to his core role as an easygoing person.

During the fifth session with Tony, I asked him to spell out in detail how his relationship with Julie would change if he was to act as if he was assertive. Tony thought that the changes may be to make things easier on himself in terms of worrying less. In addition, he said that Julie would "conform:" "She would measure up" as a result of him being in the controlling position. Finally, he added: "But I don't want to dominate." I construed Tony's response as indicating that there was still some confusion between acting assertively and taking into consideration other peoples rights as opposed to acting aggressively and neglecting others rights. When I clarified the difference, Tony said that then the relationship would still change by becoming easier for him but in addition he would gain some respect from Julie and so there would be a greater chance of getting together. At this point, I referred

Tony back to his assertive/easygoing construct and Tony replied that being easygoing was not the answer.

This in turn opened up for Tony the ways in which the relationship would change and the benefits that he construed would occur if he was to act assertively. It helped Tony reconstruct his core role in relationships. Unfortunately, I do not think the gains made here were consolidated before therapy terminated.

CONCLUSION

In summary, I conducted therapy with Tony using a variety of techniques that were chosen to help him reconstrue his constructions about himself and work and himself within his relationships. By understanding his construing a little better, it was hoped that he would integrate his cognitions with his emotions. Such goals would necessarily lead to some core role reconstruction. The techniques used were assertiveness training, providing alternative stories, elaborating his use of language, and refining construction by focusing on feelings.

In the later stage of therapy, I frequently operated within Tony's system of language and to a lesser extent his values. This permitted us to articulate some of the problematic core role structures by which he had previously organized his constructions of work and his interactions with Julie. We were able to restructure one of his major constructs having problematic consequences for his relationships: Assertive versus easygoing.

There were various obstacles that hampered therapeutic movement. Perhaps most significantly, I failed to adopt a truly open approach until later in therapy. Given that therapy lasted for only five sessions, not being sufficiently open to constructs from the onset meant that I was not making the most of the limited time we had together. My not being open enough in my approach may indicate that in personal construct terms there was not a lot of congruence in the content of our construct systems.

I found it difficult to get beyond Tony's concrete constructions of his core role in relationships. His reconstructions were therefore insufficient to provide for lasting changes in his construing and actions. Perhaps there should have been use made of enactment procedures. Enactment could have been used earlier in therapy and more roles developed as therapy progressed.

Another obstacle to therapy was Tony's isolation. Tony's isolation made it difficult for him to elaborate his construing independently of myself. Also, there was limited opportunity for Tony to have his new constructions validated outside therapy. I should have encouraged him to develop more of these opportunities.

COMMENTS FROM LINDA VINEY

This therapist has been able to use effectively the "engineering" metaphors of his client, Tony, and to help him retell his stories about work. However, he shows some lack of openness to his construing and, as a result, seems to have missed exploring his "dominance" construct. In fact, he has been rather late to elicit Tony's constructs and it is no surprise that he himself shows some confusion about the therapy. His strengths lie in the appropriateness of his self-criticisms. He has acknowledged his failure to use enactment as a way of exploring Tony's construing and he has become aware of the need for Tony to test his stories outside therapy. Most importantly, he has identified his own failure in developing stories for Tony about his relationships without sufficient input from his client.

READINGS

Adams-Webber, J.R. (1981). Fixed role therapy. In R.L. Corsini (Ed.), *Handbook of innovative psychotherapies*. New York: Wiley.

Agnew, J. (1985). Childhood disorders or the ventures of children. In E. Button (Ed.), *Personal construct theory and mental health*. London: Croom Helm.

Alexander, S., & Follette, V. (1985). Personal constructs in group treatment of incest. In R.A. Neimeyer & G.J. Neimeyer (Eds.), *Personal construct therapy casebook*. New York: Springer.

Ansbacher, H.L., & Ansbacher, R. (Eds.). (1956). *The individual psychology of Alfred Adler*. New York: Basic Books.

Arizmendi, T.G., Beutler, L.E., Shanfield, S.B., Crago, M., & Hagaman, R. (1985). Client–therapist value similarity and psychotherapy outcome: A microscopic analysis. *Psychotherapy, 22,* 16–21.

Assogioli, R. (1973). *The act of will*. Baltimore: Penguin.

Bandura, A. (1978). The self system in reciprocal determinism. *American Psychologist, 33,* 344–358.

Bannister, D., & Fransella, F. (1985). *Inquiring man*. Chichester: Wiley.

Bannister, D. (1965). The genesis of schizophrenic thought disorder: Retest of the serial invalidation hypothesis. *British Journal ofPsychiatry, 11,* 377–382.

Bannister, D. (1970a). Comment on H.J. Eysenck's explanation and the concept of personality. In R.T. Borger and F. Cioffi (Eds.), *Explanation in the behavioural sciences*. Cambridge, England: Cambridge University Press.

Bannister, D. (1970b). Science through the looking glass. In D. Bannister (Ed.), *Perspectives in personal construct theory*. London: Academic.

Bannister, D. (1975). Personal construct theory psychotherapy. In D. Bannister (Ed.), *Issues and approaches in the psychological therapies*. London: Wiley.

Bannister, D. (1983). The internal politics of psychotherapy. In D. Pilgrim (Ed.), *Psychology and psychotherapy*. London: Routledge & Kegan Paul.

Bannister, D., Adams-Webber, J.R., Penn, W.I., & Radley, A. (1975). Reversing the process of thought disorder: A serial validation experiment. *British Journal of Social and Clinical Psychology, 14,* 169–180.

Bannister, D., & Fransella, F. (1986). *Inquiring man.* Beckenham: Croom Helm.

Bannister, F., & Mair, M. (1966). *The evaluation of personal constructs.* London: Academic.

Barnes, B. (1983). Doubts and certainties in practising psychotherapy. In D. Pilgrim (Ed.), *Psychology and psychotherapy.* London: Routledge & Kegan.

Barton, A. (1971). The client-centred transformation: A phenomenological approach. In A. Giorgi, W. Fischer, & R. Von Eckartsberg (Eds.), *Duquesne studies in phenomenological psychology* (Vol. 1). Pittsburgh: Duquesne University Press.

Barton, A. (1974). *Three worlds of therapy: Freud, Jung and Rogers.* Palo Alto, CA: National Press Books.

Beail, N. (Ed.). (1985). *Repertory Grid Technique in personal construct: Applications in clinical and educational settings.* London: Croom Helm.

Beauchamp, T.L., & Childress, J.T. (1983). *Principles of biomedical ethics.* New York: Oxford University Press.

Beck, A.T. (1967). *Depression: Clinical, experimental and theoretical aspects.* New York: Harper & Row.

Beck, A.T. (1976). *Cognitive therapy and the emotional disorders.* New York: Meridian.

Beck, A.T., Emery, G., & Greenberg, R.L. (1985). *Anxiety disorders and phobias: A cognitive perspective.* New York: Basic Books.

Beck, A.T., Rush, A.J., Shaw, B.T., & Emery, G. (1979). *Cognitive therapy of depression.* New York: Guilford.

Bell, R.C. (1988). Theory appropriate analyses of Repertory Grid data. *International Journal of Personal Construct Psychology, 1,* 126–138.

Benbenishty, R., & Schul, Y. (1987). Client–therapist congruence of expectations over the course of therapy. *British Journal of Clinical Psychology, 26,* 17–24.

Berger, I.W. (1989). Developing the story in psychotherapy. *American Journal of Psychotherapy, 43,* 248–289.

Berne, E. (1964). *Games people play.* London: Penguin.

Blows, M., & Srinivasan, S. (1991). *Studies in meditation.* Melbourne: Hill of Content Press.

Blumenfied, M.D. (Ed.). (1982). *Applied supervision in psychotherapy.* New York: Grune & Stratton.

Bonarius, J.C.J. (1970). Fixed role therapy: A double paradox. *British Journal of Medical Psychology, 43,* 213–219.

Bonney, W.C., & Scott, K.U. (1983). An explanation of the origin of role formation via psychodrama and personal construct theories. *Journal of Group Psychotherapy, Psychodrama and Sociometry, 36,* 46–55.

Britton, B.K., & Pellegrini, A.D. (1990). *Narrative thought and narrative language.* Hillsdale, NJ: Erlbaum.

Burr, V.S., & Butt, T. (1992). *Invitation to personal construct psychology.* London: Shurr.

Butler, S., & Strupp, H. (1986). Specific and nonspecific factors in psychotherapy: A problematic paradigm for psychotherapy research. *Psychotherapy, 23,* 30–40.

Button, E. (Ed.). (1985). *Personal construct theory and mental health.* London: Croom Helm.
Button, E. (1992). Eating disorders and personal constructs. In R.A. Neimeyer & G.J. Neimeyer (Eds.), *Advances in personal construct psychology.* Greenwich, CT: JAI.
Button, E. (1994). *Personal construct therapy for eating disorders.* Chichester: Wiley.
Carr, D. (1985). Life and the narrator's art. In H.J. Silverman & D. Ihde (Eds.), *Hermeneutics and deconstruction.* New York: State University of New York Press.
Casement, P. (1985). *On learning from the patient.* London: Tavistock.
Catina, A., Tschuschke, V., & Winter, D. (1989). Self-reconstruction as a result of interaction in analytic group therapy. *Group Analysis, 22,* 59–62.
Chiaro, G., Nuzzo, L., Alfano, V., Brogna, P., D'Andrea, T., Di Battista, G., Plata, P., & Stefan, G. (1994). Personal paths of dependency. *International Journal of Personal Construct Psychology, 7,* 112–122.
Cochran, L. (1986). *Portrait and story: Dramaturgical approaches to the study of the person.* New York: Greenwood.
Cohen, C.D., & Cooley, S. (1983). Psychological training programs for direct services to the ageing. *Professional Psychology, 14,* 720–728.
Cohler, B.J. (1982). Personal narrative and life course. In P. Baltes & O.G. Brim (Eds.), *Life span development and behaviour* (Vol 4). New York: Academic.
Collier, A. (1977). *The philosophy and politics of psychotherapy.* Sussex: Harvester.
Combs, G., & Freedman, J. (1990). *Symbol, story and ceremony: Using metaphor in individual and family therapy.* London: Norton.
Cox, M., & Theilgaard, A. (1987). *Mutative metaphors in psychotherapy.* London: Tavistock.
Cromwell, R., Sewell, K., & Langelle, C. (1993, July). *The personal construction of trauma.* Paper presented at the 10th International Personal Construct Congress, Townsville, Australia.
Crose, R. (1990). Reviewing the past in the here and now: Using gestalt therapy techniques with life review. *Journal of Mental Health Counselling, 12,* 279–287.
Dalley, T., & Case, C. (1992). *The handbook of art therapy.* London: Routledge.
Dalton, P. (Ed.). (1980). *Approaches to the treatment of stuttering.* London: Croom Helm.
Dalton, S., & Dunnett, G. (1993). *Living personal construct psychology.* Chichester: Wiley.
Dardenne, P., & Mahtani, A. (1989). *Transcultural counselling in action.* London: Sage.
Dennett, D.C. (1983). The self as a centre of narrative gravity. In D.L. Johnson & D.M. Cole (Eds.), *Consciousness and self.* New York: Praeger.
Derlega, V.J., & Berg, J.H. (Eds.). (1987). *Self-disclosure: Theory, research and therapy.* New York: Plenum.
Dryden, W., & Trower, P. (1988). *Developments in cognitive psychotherapy.* London: Sage.

Duck, S., & Sants, H. (1983). On the origin of the species: Are interpersonal relationships really interpersonal states? *Journal of Social and Clinical Psychology, 1,* 27–41.

Dunnett, G. (1985). Construing control in theory and therapy. In D. Bannister (Ed.), *Issues and approaches in personal construct theory.* London: Academic.

Dunnett, G. (1988a). Myths, methods and techniques. In G. Dunnett (Ed.), *Working with people.* London: Routledge.

Dunnett, G. (Ed.). (1988b). *Working with people.* London: Routledge.

Eagleton T. (1983). *Literary theory.* Minneapolis: University of Minneapolis Press.

Ellis, A. (1979). Rational-emotive therapy and cognitive behaviour therapy: Similarities and differences. *Cognitive Therapy and Research, 4,* 325–340.

Ellis, A. (1984). The essence of RET–1984. *Journal of Rational-Emotive Therapy, 2,* 19–26.

Entralgo, P.L. (1970). *The therapy of the word in classical antiquity.* New Haven: Yale University Press.

Epting, F. (1981). An appraisal of personal construct psychotherapy. In H. Bonarius, R. Holland, & S. Rosenberg (Eds.), *Personal construct psychology—Recent advances in theory and practice.* London: Macmillan.

Epting, F. (1984). *Personal construct counselling and psychotherapy.* Chichester: Wiley.

Epting, F., & Amerikaner, M. (1980). Optimal functioning: A personal construct approach. In A.W. Landfield & L.M. Leitner (Eds.), *Personal construct psychology: Psychotherapy and personality.* New York: Wiley.

Epting, F.R., & Boger, P.A. (1981). Personal construct psychotherapy. In R.L. Corsini (Ed.), *Handbook of innovative psychotherapies.* New York: Wiley.

Epting, F.R., & Nazario, A. (1987). Designing a fixed role therapy: Issues, techniques and modifications. In R.A. Niemeyer & G.J. Niemeyer (Eds.), *A casebook in personal construct therapy.* New York: Springer.

Epting, F., & Neimeyer, R. A. (Eds.). (1983). *Personal meanings of death.* New York: Hemisphere.

Evesham, M., & Fransella, F. (1985). Stuttering relapse: The effects of a combined speech and psychological reconstruction program. *British Journal of Disorders of Communication, 20,* 237–248.

Fagan, N.J., & Shepherd, I.L. (1971). *Gestalt therapy now.* New York: Harper & Row.

Faidley, A.J., & Leitner, L.M. (1993). *Assessing experience in psychotherapy: Personal construct alternatives.* Westport, CT: Praeger.

Fairbairn, S., & Fairbairn, G. (1987). *Psychology, ethics and change.* London: Routledge & Kegan Paul.

Fischer, C.T. (1970). The testee as co-evaluator. *Journal of Counselling Psychology, 17,* 70–76.

Fischer, C.T. (1985). *Individualizing psychological assessment.* Monterey, CA: Brooks/Cole.

Fischer, C.T., & Fischer, W.F. (1983). Phenomenological–existential psycho-

therapy. In M. Hersen, A.E. Kazdin, & A.S. Bellack (Eds.), *The clinical psychology handbook*. New York: Pergamon.
Frank, J. (1985). Therapeutic components shared by all psychotherapies. In M.J. Mahoney & A. Freeman (Eds.), *Cognition and psychotherapy.* New York: Plenum.
Fransella, F. (1972). *Personal change and reconstruction: Research and treatment of stuttering*. London: Academic.
Fransella, F. (1981). Nature babbling to herself: The self characterization as a therapeutic tool. In H. Bonarius, R. Holland, & S. Rosenberg (Eds.), *Personal construct psychology: Recent advances in theory and in practice.* New York: St. Martin's Press.
Fransella, F. (1985). Individual psychotherapy. In E. Button, (Ed.), *Personal construct theory and mental health*. Beckenham: Croom Helm.
Fransella, F. (1987). Stuttering to fluency through reconstruction. In R.A. Neimeyer & G.J. Neimeyer (Eds.), *Personal construct therapy casebook.* New York: Springer.
Fransella, F., & Dalton, P. (1990). *Personal construct counselling in action.* London: Sage.
Freiere, P. (1972). *Peadagogy of the oppressed.* London: Pergamon.
Freud, S. (1925). *The collected papers of Sigmund Freud.* London: Hogarth.
Friedlander, M.L. (1984). Psychotherapy talk as social control. *Psychotherapy, 41,* 335–341.
Friedlander, M.L., & Schwartz, G.S. (1985). Toward a theory of strategic self-presentation in counselling and psychotherapy. *Journal of Counselling Psychology, 32,* 483–501.
Gatz, M., & Pearson, C.E. (1988). Ageism revisited and the provision of psychological services. *American Psychologist, 43,* 184–188.
Gendlin, E.T. (1981). *Focussing*. New York: Bantam.
Gendlin, E.T. (1985). *Let your body interpret your dreams*. Wilmette, IL: Chiron.
Gergen, K.J. (1985). The social constructionist movement in modern psychology. *American Psychologist, 40,* 266–275.
Gill, M. (1976). Metapsychologies not psychology. In M. Gill & P. Holzman (Eds.), Meta-psychology versus psychology: Psychoanalytic essays in memory of George S. Klein. *Psychological Issues, 9,* (Mono. 36), 210–220.
Gilligan, C. (1982). *In a different voice.* Cambridge, MA: Harvard University Press.
Gindhart, L.R. (1981). The use of a metaphoric story in therapy: A case report. *American Journal of Clinical Hypnosis, 23,* 202–206.
Goldfried, M.R. (1982). *Converging themes in psychotherapy.* New York: Springer.
Goodman, N. (1978). *Ways of world making*. New York: Harvester.
Gordon, D. (1978). *Therapeutic metaphors*. Cupertino, CA: Meta.
Gottschalk. L.A. (1985). *How to understand and analyse your own dreams.* Berkeley, CA: Arts Reproduction Press.
Granvold, D.K. (1994). *Cognitive and behavioural treatment*. Pacific Grove, CA: Brooks/Cole.

Gray, L.A., & Harding, A.K. (1988). Confidentiality limits with clients who have the AIDS virus. *Journal of Counselling and Development, 66,* 219–223.

Green, D., & Kelly-Turner, N. (1990). First steps in family therapy: A personal construct analysis. *Journal of Family Therapy, 12,* 231–250.

Guidano, U.F. (1991). *A redefinition of cognitive therapy: Using affect in the exploration of self.* New York: Guilford.

Guidano, V.F., & Liotto, G. (1985). A constructivist foundation for cognitive therapy. In M.J. Mahoney & A. Freeman (Eds.), *Cognition and psychotherapy.* New York: Plenum.

Harter, S., Alexander, P.C., & Neimeyer, R.A. (1988). Long term effects of incestuous child abuse in college women: Social adjustment, social cognition and family characteristics. *Journal of Consulting & Clinical Psychology, 56,* 5–8.

Hayhow, R., & Levy, C. (1989). *Working with stuttering: A personal construct approach.* Bicester, England: Winslow Press.

Hermans, H.J.M., Kempen, H.J.G., & Van Loon, R.J.P. (1992). The dialogical self: Beyond individualism and rationalism. *American Psychologist, 47,* 23–32.

Hess, A.K. (Ed.). (1980). *Psychotherapy supervision: Theory, research and practice.* Chichester: Wiley.

Hobson, R.F. (1985). *Forms of feeling.* London: Tavistock.

Hoffman, L. (1992). A reflexive stance for family therapy. In S. McNamee & K. Gergen (Eds.), *Therapy as a social construction.* Newbury Park, CA: Sage.

Holland, R. (1970). George Kelly: Constructive innocent and reluctant existensialist. In D. Bannister (Ed.), *Perspectives in personal construct theory.* London: Academic.

Hoshmand, L.T. (1993). The personal narrative in the construction of self and life issues. In G.J. Neimeyer (Ed.), *Constructivist assessment: A casebook.* New York: Sage.

Jackson, S. (1990). A personal construct therapy group for adolescents. In P. Maitland (Ed.), *Personal construct theory deviancy and social work.* London: Centre for Personal Construct Psychology.

Jennings, J.L. (1986). Husserl revisited: The forgotten distinction between psychology and phenomenology. *American Psychologist, 41,* 1231–1240.

Jennings, S. (1987). *Drama therapy.* London: Routledge.

Joyce-Moniz, L. (1985). Epistemological therapy and constructivism. In M.J. Mahoney & A. Freeman (Eds.), *Cognition and psychotherapy.* New York: Plenum.

Kain, C.D. (1988). To breach or not breach: Is that the question? A response to Gray and Harding. *Journal of Counselling and Development, 68,* 224–225.

Kalekin-Fischmann, D., & Walker, B. (1995). *The construction of group realities. Culture, society and personal construct theory.* Melbourne, FL: Krieger.

Karst, T.O., & Trexler, L.D. (1974). Initial study using fixed role and rational-emotive therapy in treating speaking anxiety. *Journal of Consulting and Clinical Psychology, 34,* 360–366.

Katakis, C.D. (1989). Stages of psychotherapy: Progressive reconceptualizations as a self-organizing process. *Psychotherapy, 26,* 462–468.

Keating, D.P., & Rosen, H. (1991). *Constructivist perspectives on developmental psychopathology and atypical development.* Hillsdale, NJ: Erlbaum.

Keen, E. (1972). *Psychology and the new consciousness.* Monterey, CA: Brooks/Cole.

Keen, E. (1977). Existensial–phenomenological therapy. In D. Rimm & J.W. Somervill (Eds.), *Abnormal psychology.* New York: Academic.

Kelly, G.A. (1955). *The psychology of personal constructs.* New York: Norton.

Kelly, G.A. (1964). The language of hypothesis: Man's psychological instrument. *Journal of Individual Psychology, 20,* 137–152.

Kelly, G.A. (1967). A psychology of the optimal man. In A.H. Mahrer (Ed.), *The goals of psychotherapy.* New York: Appleton-Century-Crofts.

Kelly, G.A. (1969a). Epilogue: Don Juan. In B. Maher (Ed.), *Clinical psychology and personality.* New York: Wiley.

Kelly, G.A. (1969b). In whom confide: On whom depend for what? In B. Maher (Ed.), *Clinical psychology and personality.* New York: Wiley.

Kelly, G.A. (1989). *The function of interpretation in psychotherapy: Techniques of psychotherapeutic reinterpretation.* London: The Centre for Personal Construct Psychology.

Kendall, P.C. (Ed.). (1985). *Advances in cognitive-behavioural research and therapy.* New York: Academic.

Kenny, J. (1987). Autopoesis and alternativisim in psychotherapy: Fluctuations and reconstructions. In F. Fransella & L. Thomas (Eds.), *Experimenting with personal construct psychology.* London: Routledge & Kegan Paul.

Kenny, J. (1988). Changing conversations: A constructivist model of training for psychotherapists. In G. Dunnett (Ed.), *Working with people: Clinical uses of personal construct psychology.* London: Routledge.

Klein, G. (1976). *Psychoanalytic theory.* New York: International Universities Press.

Koch, H. (1985). Group psychotherapy. In E. Button (Ed.), *Personal construct theory and mental health.* Beckenham: Croom Helm.

Koch, H.C.H. (1983). Changes in personal construing in the psychotherapy group and a control group. *British Journal of Medical Psychology, 56,* 245–255.

Kuhlman, T.L. (1984). *Humour and psychotherapy.* Homewood, IL: Dorsey Press.

Kurtzman, H.S. (1987). Deconstruction and psychology: An introduction. *New Ideas in Psychology, 5,* 33–71.

Lakin, M. (1991). *Coping with ethical dilemmas in psychotherapy.* Elmsford, NY: Pergamon.

Lakoff, G., & Johnson, M. (1980). *Metaphors we live by.* Chicago: University of Chicago Press.

Lamiell, J.I. (1987). *The psychology of personality: An epistemological enquiry.* New York: Columbia University Press.

Landfield, A.W. (1971). *Personal construct systems in psychotherapy.* Chicago: Rand McNally.

Landfield, A.W. (1984). Personal construct psychology: A developmental perspective. *Journal of Social & Clinical Psychology, 2,* 97–107.

Landfield, A.W., & Epting, F.R. (1987). *Personal construct psychology: Clinical personality assessment.* New York: Human Sciences.

Landfield, A.W., & Rivers, P.C. (1975). An introduction to interpersonal transaction and rotating dyads. *Psychotherapy, 12,* 366–374.

Lawless, D.J. (1989). Religious values in the workplace. *Organisational Development Journal, 11,* 1–9.

Leitner, L., & Guthrie, A.J. (1993). Validation of therapist interventions in psychotherapy: Clarity ambiguity and subjectivity. *International Journal of Personal Construct Psychology, 6,* 281–294.

Leitner, L.M. (1985a). Interview methodologies for construct elicitation: Searching for the core. In F. Epting & A.W. Landfield (Eds.), *Anticipating personal construct psychology.* Lincoln: University of Nebraska Press.

Leitner, L.M. (1985b). The terrors of cognition: On the experiential validity of personal construct theory. In D. Bannister (Ed.), *Issues and approaches in personal construct theory.* London: Academic.

Leitner, L.M. (1988). Terror, risk and reverence: Experiential personal construct psychotherapy. *International Journal of Personal Construct Psychology, 1,* 251–262.

Leitner, L.M., & Dill-Standiford, T. (1993). Resistance in experiential personal construct psychotherapy: Theoretical and technical struggles. In L.M. Leitner & G. Dunnet (Eds.), *Critical issues in personal construct psychology.* Malabar, FL: Krieger.

Leitner, L.M., & Pfenninger, D.T. (1994). Sociality and optimal functioning. *Journal of Constructivist Psychology, 7,* 119–136.

Lincoln, Y.S. (1990). The working of a constructivist: A remembrance of transformations past. In E.G. Guba (Ed.), *The paradigm dialogue.* London: Sage.

Llewelyn, S., & Dunnett, G. (1987). The use of personal construct theory in groups. In R.A. Neimeyer & G.J. Neimeyer (Eds), *Personal construct theory casebook.* New York: Springer.

Mahoney, M.J. (1988a). Constructivist metatheory: I. Basic features and historical foundations. *International Journal of Personal Construct Psychology, 1,* 1–36 .

Mahoney, M.J. (1988b). Constructivist metatheory: II. Implications for psychotherapy. *Journal of Personal Construct Psychology, 1,* 299–316.

Mahoney, M.J., & Freeman, A. (Eds.). (1985). *Cognition and psychotherapy.* New York: Plenum.

Mahoney, M.J., & Gabriel, T.J. (1987). Psychotherapy and the cognitive sciences: An evolving alliance. *Journal of Cognitive Psychotherapy, 1,* 39–59.

Mahoney, M.J., & Lydon, W.J. (1988). Recent developments in cognitive approaches to counselling and psychotherapy. *The Counselling Psychologist, 16,* 190–234.

Mahoney, M.J. (1995). The psychological demands of being a constructivist therapist. In R.A. Neimeyer & M.J. Mahoney (Eds.), *Constructivism in psychotherapy.* Washington, D.C.: American Psychological Association.

Mahrer, A.H. (1985). *Psychotherapeutic change.* New York: Norton.

Mahrer, A.H. (1986). *Therapeutic experiencing.* New York: Norton.

Mahrer, A.H. (1992). *The integration of psychotherapies.* New York: Human Sciences.

Mair, J.M.M. (1976). Metaphors for living. *Nebraska Symposium on Motivation, 24,* 243–290.

Mair, J.M.M. (1988a). George Kelly, Don Bannister and a story-telling psychology. *International Journal of Personal Construct Psychology, 2,* 1–14.

Mair, J.M.M. (1988b). Psychology as story telling. *International Journal of Personal Construct Psychology, 1,* 125–137.

Mair, J.M.M. (1989). *Between psychology and psychotherapy: A poetry of experience.* London: Routledge.

Mair, J.M.M. (1990). Telling psychological tales. *International Journal of Personal Construct Psychology, 3,* 1–22.

Maitland, P. X.X. (Ed.). (1990). *Personal construct theory, deviancy and social work.* London: Inner London Probation Service and the Centre for Personal Construct Psychology.

Mancuso, J.C. (1979). Counselling from a personal construct perspective. *International Journal for the Advancement of Counselling, 110,* 305–313.

Markova, I. (1987). *Paradigms, thought and language.* Chichester: Wiley.

Mascolo, M. (1994). Towards a social constructivist psychology: The case of self-evaluative emotional development. *Journal of Constructivist Psychology, 7,* 107–119.

May, R. (1964). On the phenomenological bases of psychotherapy. *Review of Existensial Psychology and Psychiatry, 4,* 22–36.

May, R. (Ed.). (1969). *Existensial psychology.* New York: Random House.

McAdams, D.P. (1985). *Power, intimacy and the life story.* Homewood, IL: Dorsey Press.

McCoy, M. (1980). Positive and negative emotion: A personal construct theory interpretation. In H. Bonarius, R.S.Holland, & S. Rosenberg (Eds.), *Recent advances in the theory and practice of personal construct psychology.* London: Macmillan.

McKain, T.L., Glass, C.R., Arnkoff, D.D., Sydnor-Greenberg, J.M., & Shea, C.A. (1988). Personal constructs and shyness: The relationship between Repertory Grid data and therapy outcome. *International Journal of Personal Construct Psychology, 1,* 151–167.

McNamee, S., & Gergen, K.J. (Eds.). (1992). *Therapy as social construction.* New York: Plenum.

Meltzer, D. (1978). *The Kleinian development.* Strath Tay, Perthshire: Clunie Press.

Mental Health Task Force. (1991). *Mental health: A statement of rights and responsibilities.* Canberra: Australian Government Printing Service.

Miall, D.S. (1989). Anticipating the self: Towards a personal construct construct model of emotion. *International Journal of Personal Construct Psychology, 2,* 185–198.

Mills, J.C., & Crowley, R.J. (1986). *Therapeutic metaphors for children and the child within*. New York: Brunner/Mazel.

Mintz, J., Auerbach, A.H., Luborsky, L., & Johnson, M. (1973). Patients', therapists' and observers' views of psychotherapy: A Rashomon experience or a reasonable consensus? *British Journal of Medical Psychology, 46,* 85–89.

Mischel, W. (1980). George Kelly's anticipation of psychology: A personal tribute. In M.J. Mahoney (Ed.), *Psychotherapy process*. New York: Plenum.

Murphy, G.L., & Medin, D.L. (1985). The role of theories in conceptual coherence. *Psychological Review, 92,* 289–316.

Nash, C. (Ed.). (1990). *Narrative in culture*. New York: Routledge, Chapman & Hall.

Neimeyer, G.J. (1987). Personal construct assessment, strategy and technique. In R.A. Neimeyer & G.J. Neimeyer (Eds.), *Personal construct therapy casebook*. New York: Springer.

Neimeyer, G.J. (Ed.). (1993). *Constructivist assessment: A casebook*. New York: Sage.

Neimeyer, G.J., & Merluzzi, T.V. (1991). Group structure and group process: Explorations in therapeutic sociality. *Small Group Behaviour, 13,* 150–164.

Neimeyer, G.J., & Neimeyer, R.A. (1993). Defining the boundaries of constructivist assessment. In G.J. Neimeyer (Ed.), *Constructivist assessment*. New York: Sage.

Neimeyer, R.A. (1985). Personal constructs in clinical practice. In P.C. Kendall (Ed.), *Advances in cognitive-behavioural research and therapy*. New York: Academic.

Neimeyer, R.A. (1986). Personal construct therapy. In W. Dryden & W.L. Golden (Eds.), *Cognitive-behavioural approaches to psychotherapy*. London: Harper & Row.

Neimeyer, R.A. (1988). Clinical guide-lines for conducting Interpersonal Transaction Groups. *International Journal of Personal Construct Psychology, 1,* 181–190.

Neimeyer, R.A. (1993a). An appraisal of constructivist psychotherapies. *Journal of Consulting and Clinical Psychology, 61,* 221–234.

Neimeyer, R.A. (1993b). Constructivist approaches to the measurement of meaning. In G.J. Neimeyer (Ed.), *Constructivist assessment: A casebook*. New York: Sage.

Neimeyer, R.A. (1995). Constructivist psychotherapies: Features, foundations and future directions. In R.A. Neimeyer & M.J. Mahoney (Eds.), *Constructivism in psychotherapy*. Washington, D.C.: American Psychological Association.

Neimeyer, R.A., & Epting, F.R. (1992). Measuring personal meanings of death: Twenty years of research using the Threat Index. In R.A. Neimeyer & G.J. Neimeyer (Eds.), *Advances in personal construct psychology*. Greenwich, CT: JAI.

Neimeyer, R.A., & Harter, S. (1988). Facilitating individual change in personal construct therapy. In G. Dunnett (Ed.), *Personal construct psychology in clinical settings*. London: Routledge & Kegan Paul.

Neimeyer, R.A., & Neimeyer, G.J. (1983). Structural similarity in the acquaintance process. *Journal of Social and Clinical Psychology, 1,* 146–154.

Neimeyer, R.A., & Neimeyer, G.J. (1985). Disturbed relationships: A personal construct view. In E. Button (Ed.), *Personal construct theory and mental health*. Beckenham: Croom Helm.

Papanek, H. (1964). Bridging dichotomies through group psychotherapy. *Journal of Individual Psychology, 20,* 38–47.

Pentony, P. (1981). *Models of influence in psychotherapy.* London: Collier Macmillan.

Pilgrim, D. (Ed.). (1983). *Psychology and psychotherapy.* London: Routledge & Kegan Paul.

Polanyi, M., & Prosch, H. (1975). *Meaning*. Chicago: University of Chicago Press.

Polster, E. (1985). Escape from the present: Transitions and story line. In J. Zeig (Ed.), *The evaluation of psychotherapy.* New York: Brunner/Mazel.

Polster, E. (1987). *Every person's life is worth a novel.* New York: Norton.

Pope, K.S. (1990). Therapist–patient sexual involvement: A review of the research. *Clinical Psychology Review, 10,* 477–490.

Popper, K.R. (1989). *The logic of scientific discovery.* New York: Basic Books.

Proctor, H. (1981). Family construct psychology: An approach to understanding and treating families. In S. Walrond-Skinner (Ed.), *Developments in family therapy.* London: Routledge & Kegan Paul.

Quattrone, G.A. (1985). On the congruity between internal states and actions. *Psychological Bulletin, 98,* 3–40.

Rabbitt, P., & Abson, J. (1991). Do older people know how good they are? *British Journal of Psychology, 82,* 132–151.

Ravenette, A.T. (1993, July). *Asking questions within a personal construct framework.* Paper presented at the 10th International Personal Construct Congress, Townsville, Australia.

Rogers, C.R. (1959). A theory of therapy, personality and interpersonal relationships as developed in a client-centered framework. In S. Koch (Ed.), *Psychology: A study of a science.* New York: McGraw-Hill.

Romanyshyn, R.D. (1982). *Psychological life: From science to metaphor.* Milton Keynes: The Open University.

Ross, M.W. (1989). Psychosocial ethical aspects of AIDS. *Journal of Medical Ethics, 15,* 74–81.

Rowe, D. (1989). *Depression: The way out of your prison.* London: Routledge.

Rubin, J.A. (1987). *Approaches to art therapy.* New York: Brunner/Mazel.

Rubin, R.J. (Ed.). (1978). *Bibliotherapy sourcebook.* Phoenix: Onyx.

Rudestam, K.E. (1980). *Methods of self change.* Belmont, CA: Brooks/Cole.

Rychlak, J.F. (1968). *A philosophy of science of personality.* Boston: Houghton Mifflin.

Rychlak, J.F. (1981). *Introduction to personality and psychotherapy.* Boston: Houghton Mifflin.

Rychlak, J.F. (1982). Some therapeutic implications of logical phenomenology. *Psychotherapy, 19,* 259–265.

Rychlak, J.F. (1983). Exclusivity in psychological specialization: A conceptual or practical problem? *Journal of Social & Clinical Psychology, 1,* 185–192.
Ryle, A. (1992). *A cognitive psychotherapy.* London: Sage.
Ryle, A., & Lipshitz, S. (1976). An intensive case study of a therapeutic group. *British Journal of Psychiatry, 128,* 581–587.
Salmon, P. (1980). *Coming to know.* London: Routledge & Kegan Paul.
Saper, B. (1987). Humour as psychotherapy: Is it good or bad for the client? *Professional Psychology: Research and Practise, 18,* 360–367.
Sarbin,T. (Ed.). (1986). *Narrative psychology: The shared nature of human conduct.* New York: Praeger.
Schacht, T.E., & Black, D.A. (1985). Epistemological commitments of behavioural and psychoanalytic therapists. *Professional Psychology: Research and Practice, 16,* 316–323.
Schafer, R. (1980). Narration in the psychoanalytic dialogue. *Critical Enquiry, 7,* 29–53.
Schafer, R. (1983). *The analytic attitude.* New York: Basic Books.
Schmidt, J. (1984). Counsellor intentionality: An emerging view of process and performance. *Journal of Counselling Psychology, 31,* 383–386.
Schütz, A. (1972). *Phenomenology of the social world.* London: Heineman.
Schwartz, G.S., Friedlander, M.L., & Tedeschi, J.T. (1986). Effects of clients' attributional explanations and reasons for seeking help on counsellors' impressions. *Journal of Counselling Psychology, 33,* 90–93.
Shainberg, D. (1980). The relationship of theory to therapy. *Comprehensive Psychotherapy, 1,* 93–110.
Shapiro, T. (1979). *Clinical psycholinguistics.* London: Plenum.
Sheehan, W.J. (1985). A personal construct study of depression. *British Journal of Medical Psychology, 72,* 197–209.
Siegelman, E.Y. (1990). *Metaphor and meaning in psychotherapy.* New York: Guilford.
Silberschazz, G., Curtis, J.T., & Nathan, S. (1989). Using the patient's plan to assess progress in psychotherapy. *Psychotherapy, 26,* 40–46.
Simon, R. (1988, September–October). The constructivist challenge: An interview with Lyn Hoffman. *Networker,* 55–59.
Skene, R.A. (1973). Construct shift in the treatment of a case of homosexuality. *British Journal of Medical Psychology, 46,* 287–288.
Smith, D.L. (1979). Phenomenological psychotherapy: A why and how. In A. Giorgi, R. Knowles, & D.L. Smith (Eds.), *Duquesne studies in phenomenological psychology* (Vol. 3). Pittsburgh: Duquesne University Press.
Soldz, S. (1988). Constructivist tendencies in recent psychoanalysis. *International Journal of Personal Construct Psychology, 1,* 329–348.
Spinelli, L. (1989). *The interpreted world.* London: Sage.
Steiner, M., Newall, J.D., & Garcia, C.T. (1984). *Ethical issues in psychology.* Homewood, IL: Dorsey Press.
Strohmer, D.C., & Chiodo, A.L. (1984). Counsellor hypothesis testing strategies: The role of initial impressions and self schema. *Journal of Counselling Psychology, 31,* 510–519.

Sue, D.W. (1981). *Counselling the culturally different.* New York: Wiley.
Thompson, M. (1989). *On art and therapy.* London: Virago Press.
Tracey, T.J., Heck, E.J., & Lichtenberg, J.W. (1981). Role expectations and symmetrical/complementary therapeutic relationships. *Psychotherapy, 18,* 338–344.
Vaihinger, H. (1911). *The philosophy of as if.* Berlin: Reuter & Reuter.
Van den Berg, J.H. (1971). What is psychotherapy? *Humanitas, 7,* 321–370.
Viney, L.L. (1981). Experimenting with experience: A psychotherapeutic case study. *Psychotherapy, 18,* 271–278.
Viney, L.L. (1985a). Humour as a therapeutic tool. In A. Landfield & F. Epting (Eds.), *Anticipating personal construct theory.* Lincoln: University of Nebraska Press.
Viney, L.L. (1985b). Physical illness: A guidebook for the kingdom of the sick. In E. Button (Ed.), *Personal construct theory and mental health.* Beckenham: Croom Helm.
Viney, L.L. (1987a). *Interpreting the interpreters: Strategies for a science of construing people.* Malabar, FL: Krieger.
Viney, L.L. (1987b). A sociophenomenological approach to life span development complementing Erikson's psychodynamic approach. *Human Development, 30,* 125–136.
Viney, L.L. (1988). Psychotherapy as reconstruction. *International Journal of Personal Construct Psychology, 1,* 30–51.
Viney, L.L. (1989). *Images of illness.* Melbourne, FL: Krieger.
Viney, L.L. (1990a). A constructivist model of psychological reactions to illness and injury. In G.J. Neimeyer & R.A. Neimeyer (Eds.), *Advances in personal construct psychology* (Vol. 1). New York: JAI.
Viney, L.L. (1990b). The construing widow: Dislocation and adaptation in bereavement. *Psychotherapy Patient, 3,* 207–222.
Viney, L.L. (1992). Can we see ourselves changing?: Toward a constructivist model of adult lifespan development. *Human Development, 36,* 65–75.
Viney, L.L. (in press). A constructivist model of crisis intervention counselling. *Journal of Constructivist Psychology.*
Viney, L.L. (1993b). Goals in psychotherapy: Some reflections of a constructivist therapist. In L. Leitner & G. Dunnett (Eds.), *Critical issues in personal construct therapy.* Malabar, FL: Krieger.
Viney, L.L. (1993c). The goals of reconstructive therapy: Reflections of a therapist. In G. Dunnett & L. Leitner (Eds.), *Critical issues in personal construct therapy.* Malabar, FL: Krieger.
Viney, L.L. (1993d). *Life stories: Personal construct therapy for the elderly.* Chichester: Wiley.
Viney, L.L. (1993e). Listening to what my clients say: Content analysis categories and scales. In G.J. Neimeyer (Ed.), *Casebook of constructivist assessment.* New York: Sage.
Viney, L.L. (1994). Reminiscence in psychotherapy with the elderly: Telling and retelling their stories. In B.K. Haight & J.D. Webster (Eds.), *The art and science of reminiscing.* New York: Taylor & Francis.
Viney, L.L. (1994). Sequences of emotional distress expressed by clients and

acknowledged by therapists. *British Journal of Clinical Psychology, 33,* 469–481.

Viney, L.L., Allwood, K., & Stillson, L. (1991). Reconstructive group therapy for HIV seropositive patients. *Counselling Psychology Quarterly, 4,* 243–254.

Viney, L.L., Allwood, K., Stillson, L., & Walmsley, R. (1992a). Caring for the carers: A note on counselling for the wider impact of AIDS. *Journal of Counselling and Psychological Development, 70,* 441–446.

Viney, L.L., Allwood, K., Stillson, L., & Walmsley, R. (1992b). Personal construct therapy for clients who are HIV antibody positive. *Psychotherapy, 29,* 430–437.

Viney, L.L., Benjamin, Y.N., & Preston, C. (1988). Family therapy for the elderly: A personal construct perspective. *Journal of Family Psychology, 2,* 39–48.

Viney, L.L., Benjamin, Y.N., & Preston, C. (1988–1989). Mourning and reminiscence: Parallel psychotherapeutic processes for the elderly. *International Journal for Ageing and Human Development, 18,* 237–249.

Viney, L.L., Benjamin, Y.N., & Preston, C.A. (1989). An evaluation of personal construct therapy for the elderly. *British Journal of Medical Psychology, 62,* 35–41.

Viney, L.L., Benjamin, Y.N., & Preston, C. (1990). Personal construct therapy for the elderly. *International Journal of Cognitive Therapy, 4,* 211–224.

Viney, L.L., Benjamin, Y.N., & Preston, C. (1992). Personal construct therapy for the elderly. *International Journal of Cognitive Therapy, 4,* 26–35.

Viney, L.L., & Bousfield, L. (1993). AIDS and the client "in the fast lane": Narrative construction and reconstruction. *Psychotherapy Patient, 6,* 141–156.

Viney, L.L., Clarke, A.M., Bunn, T.A., & Benjamin, Y.N. (1985a). Crisis intervention counselling: An evaluation of long-term and short-term effects. *Journal of Counselling Psychology, 32,* 29–39.

Viney, L.L., Clarke, A.M., Bunn, T.A., & Benjamin, Y.N. (1985b). The effects of a hospital-based counselling service on the physical recovery of surgical and medical patients. *General Hospital Psychiatry, 7,* 294–301.

Viney, L.L., Truneckova, D., Weekes, P., & Oades, L. (1994, September). *Personal construct group therapy for adolescents.* Paper presented at the Australian Psychological Society Conference, Wollongong.

Viney, L.L., Walker, B., & Crooks, L. (1995). Anxiety in community-based AIDS care givers before and after counselling. *Journal of Clinical Psychology, 51,* 201–217.

Warner, R. (1976–1977). The relationship between language and disease concepts. *International Journal of Psychiatry in Medicine, 7,* 57–78.

Watzlawick, P. (1990). *Munchausen's pigtail.* London: Norton.

Webster, J.D., & Cappeliez, P. (1993). Reminiscence and autobiographical memory: Complimentary contexts for cognitive aging research. *Developmental Review, 13,* 54–91.

Weiss, J., Sampson, H., & The Mount Zion Psychotherapy Research Group. (1986). *The psychoanalytic process.* New York: Guilford.

White, M., & Epson, D. (1990). *Narrative means to therapeutic ends.* London: Norton.

Winefield, H.R., Bassett, D.L., Chandler, M., & Proske, I. (1987). Process in psychotherapy as decreasing asymmetry between patient and therapist: Evidence from the verbal interaction. *American Journal of Psychotherapy, 41,* 117–126.

Winter, D. (1988a). PCP: A radical alternative to social skills training. In P. Maitland (Ed.), *Personal construct theory, deviancy and social work.* London: Inner London Probation Service and the Centre for Personal Construct Psychology.

Winter, D.A. (1988b). Reconstruing an erection and elaborating ejaculation: Personal construct theory perspective on sex. *International Journal of Personal Construct Psychology, 1,* 81–100.

Winter, D. (1988c). Towards a constructive clinical psychology. In G. Dunnett (Ed.), *Working with people.* London: Routledge.

Winter, D.A. (1990). Therapeutic alternatives for psychological disorder: Personal construct psychology investigations in a health service setting. In G.J. Neimeyer & R.A. Neimeyer (Eds.), *Advances in personal construct psychology.* New York: JAI.

Winter, D. (1992). *Personal construct psychology in clinical practice.* London: Routledge.

Winter, D.A., & Trippett, C.J. (1977). Serial change in group psychotherapy. *British Journal of Medical Psychology, 50,* 341–348.

Witzum, E., Hart, O., & Friedman, B. (1989). The use of metaphors in psychotherapy. *Journal of Contemporary Psychotherapy, 18,* 270–290.

Wolpe, J.P. (1969). *The practice of behaviour therapy.* Elmsford, NY: Pergamon.

Woodfield, R.L., & Viney, L.L. (1985). A personal construct approach to bereavement. *Omega, 16,* 1–13.

Worden, W. (1991). *Grief counselling and grief therapy.* London: Routledge.

World Health Organization. (1981). *Global strategy for health for all by the year 2000.* Geneva: Author.

Yablonsky, L. (1981). *Psychodrama.* New York: Gardner.

Yalom, I. (1985). *The theory and practice of group psychotherapy.* New York: Basic Books.

Zeig, J. (1983). Erickson's use of anecdotes. In J. Zeig (Ed.), *A teaching seminar with Milton Erickson M.D.* New York: Brunner/Mazel.

GLOSSARY

Abstraction

In abstraction, people's approaches to their worlds become more general, less related to the physical world, and have a higher level of conceptualization.

Adaptation of Construing

When people face major losses, they can adapt their construing either by changing to new sources of confirmation or to new constructs with which to make sense of events.

Anger

Anger is experienced when people get no confirmation for their predictions about events and try to extract some.

Anxiety

Anxiety is experienced when people become aware that they do not have the constructs to make the interpretations and predictions about events that they need.

Awareness, levels of

People's levels of awareness vary from low to high. Low levels of awareness are likely when their expressed meanings are unusual or they have difficulty putting them into words. High levels are suggested by verbal account of events that are easily shared with others.

Bipolar Constructs

When constructs are used, they imply that both similarities and differences are perceived between events. They are therefore bipolar, providing a choice between two opposing predictions and courses of actions.

Commonality of Construing

The constructs that people share have commonality.

Concretization

In concretization, peoples' approaches to their worlds become more specific, more related to the physical world, and have a lower level of conceptualization.

Constriction

Constriction occurs when people reduce the number of events with which they deal because of apparent incongruity between them.

Constructs

These are the meanings by which people make sense of their lives. They are interpretations that aid in understanding the past and present and predicting the future. They are based on comparisons of events in terms of their similarities and differences.

Construct Systems

In construct systems, people's constructs are recognized as influencing one another and being influenced.

Construction

The application of constructs to make sense of one's world constitutes construction.

Constructive Alternativism

There are as many ways to make sense of the world as there are people to make sense of it.

Constructivism

Constructivism involves a set of assumptions about the nature of the world, which maintains that any account of that world must be constrained by the constructions or creations of the people who devised that account.

Constructivist Psychology

A constructivist psychology is one that maintains that, in order to understand people, their created and shared meanings must be understood. It also views that psychological understanding as a product of the shared meanings of psychologists.

Construing

Construing involves making sense of present and past events and making predictions about those in the future.

Counter Transference

Counter transference refers to the transfer of early stories about oneself by the therapist to events in therapy, without retesting their predictive value there.

Core Constructs

Constructs that are referred to as core are those by which we make sense of our selves, which are the most central, stable, and sustaining.

Core Role Constructs

Core role constructs are the most central, stable, and identity-sustaining constructs people use for predicting their interactions with others.

Creativity Cycle

The creativity cycle is used to make sense of new situations. It starts with open-ended construing and ends with construing that is more precise and useful for decision making.

Dependency, Dispersed

When people see themselves as using help from a wide range of people, their dependencies are dispersed.

Dependency, Undispersed

When people see themselves as using help from only a narrow range of people, their dependencies are undispersed.

Dialogue, Constructive

Psychotherapy occurs in two-way interactions between client and therapist during which they interpret, individually and together, what happens.

Dialogue, Reconstructive

Psychotherapy occurs in two-way interaction between client and therapist during which they reinterpret, individually and together, what happens.

Dilation

Dilation occurs when people expand the number of events of that they make sense that has the effect of expanding the range of application of their constructs.

Dislocation of Construing

When people face major losses, their construing may be dislocated so that they temporarily fail to predict events well.

Emotions

Emotions vary with people's success in interpreting their worlds. When their interpretation is effective, they experience positive emotions but when it is not, they experience negative emotions.

Enactment

Enactment involves acting out particular events (or relationships) to encourage reconstruing of those events and to develop new courses of actions.

Fixed-Role Therapy

Fixed-role therapy involves clients in acting out specific roles designed by therapists but using clients' constructs.

Goals

Goals are projects that people plan to accomplish.

Guilt

Guilt arises with awareness that one's actions do not fit with one's most central constructs about oneself.

Hostility

Hostility is experienced when people try vigorously to confirm their disconfirmed interpretations and predictions.

Impermeability

Construing has impermeability if it cannot be applied to new events and people.

Insight

Insight involves the effective use of constructs by people for interpreting and predicting their own actions.

Invalidation

When people's predictions of events, which they have based on their construing, are disconfirmed, distressing emotions result.

Laddering

Laddering involves asking the question "why?" in order to discover the more abstract and influential implications of the meanings people use.

Language

The term *language* is used here to refer not to those that are culturally based, but to the choice of words within those languages in which people speak of events.

Life Span

This is the period in people's lives, from infancy to old age, during which they continually interpret and reinterpret the events they experience.

Loose Construing

Construing that is loose leads to predictions about events that can change but are recognizably related to each other.

Metaphor

To use metaphor is to deal with one event in terms of another often similar to it in order to explore the many possible meanings of that event.

Myths

Myths are stories based on little confirmation from experienced events. They are often shared by groups of people.

Narratives

Narratives are stories in which events or constructs are integrated. They provide order and meaning in people's lives. The terms *narrative* and *story* are interchangeable.

Objectivity

An objective psychology is one that views people from a predominantly external and relatively impersonal perspective.

Openness

Therapists who are open to their clients attend to their meanings and see events from their clients' vantage points.

Permeability

Construing has permeability if it can be applied readily to new events or people.

Personal Construct Psychologyo

This is a constructivist theory developed by George Kelly.

Personal Construct Therapy

This is a constructivist psychotherapy developed by George Kelly.

Phenomenology

Phenomenology is a philosophy that involves a set of assumptions about the world that maintains that all knowledge of it is personal knowledge. It includes some techniques for detecting and controlling the role of personal meanings in developing views of that world.

Preverbal Construing

Construing that is preverbal takes place even when there are no words with which to talk about it.

Project

Projects are purposes or goals people want or intend to achieve. In therapy, they are shared by clients and therapists, although they are often for clients.

Propositionality

Construing has propositionality if it implies only the predictions related to the specific construct referred to. It is relatively uncontaminated by other constructs.

Psychosis

This is a diagnostic term applied by nonconstructivists to people who are psychologically fragile. In constructivist terms, this fragility usually implies a history of invalidation and continuing fear and avoidance of close relationships with others.

Pyramiding

Pyramiding involves asking the questions of "How?" or "What?" in order to discover the more concrete and specific implications of the meanings people use.

Reconstruction

Any reinterpretation of the meaning of events is reconstruction.

Reconstructive Therapy

In reconstructive therapy, clients and therapists together revise some important meanings of those clients and retell their stories.

Reflection

Reflection requires being aware of one's own role in interpreting events.

Reflexivity

Reflexivity involves using any psychological theory to account for its theorist as well as other people. Of reconstructive therapy, it requires that therapists be accounted for using the concepts employed for clients.

Repertory Grid Techniques

Repertory Grid Techniques are used for assessing the content of people's personal meanings and how they use them. They were developed from personal construct theory.

Role Relationships

Role relationships are relationships between people in which each participant tries to take the perspective of the other.

Self-Characterization

Self-characterization is a simple personal construct theory technique for assessing the content of people's personal meanings.

Slot Rattling

Clients may try changing their construing by using the opposite construct pole to that which they prefer. Of course, this results in no lasting change in their actions because it involves no change in their constructs.

Stories

Stories are narratives in which events or constructs are integrated. They provide order and meaning in peoples' lives. The terms *story* and *narrative* are interchangeable.

Subjectivity

A subjective psychology is one that views people from a predominantly internal and personal perspective.

Subordinacy

Subordinate constructs are lower order constructs in the hierarchical system of constructs that are influenced by and understood through other constructs.

Subsuming System of Constructs

A subsuming system of constructs can enable its user, usually a therapist, to attend to and work with another construct system without being overwhelmed by it. Therapists need to develop such systems.

Superordinacy

Superordinate constructs are higher order constructs in the hierarchical system of constructs that influence and can be used to understand other constructs.

Transference

Transference refers to the transfer of early stories about oneself and events to new events, without retesting their value as predictors.

Traumatic Stress Disorder

This is another diagnostic term, not often used by constructivists, to describe the long-term severely debilitating psychological reaction of people to threat. Natural disasters, like earthquakes, and personal disasters, like rape, can lead to this reaction.

Threat

People experience threat when they recognize the imminent possibility of major changes to their most central constructs about self.

Tight Construing

Construing that is tight leads to unvarying predictions about events.

Validation

When people's predictions about events, which they have based on their construing, are confirmed, enjoyable emotions occur.

Author Index

Subject Index

www.ingramcontent.com/pod-product-compliance
Ingram Content Group UK Ltd.
Pitfield, Milton Keynes, MK11 3LW, UK
UKHW020804290926
15470UKWH00003B/952

9 781567 50229